Making the Transition to Home Health Nursing

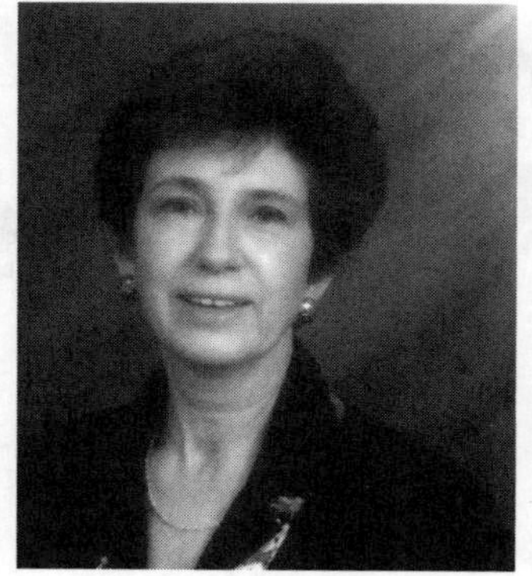

Denise Lovejoy, RN, MS, received her diploma in nursing from Laval University in Canada and her BS and MS from Columbia Pacific University in California. During her nursing career she has held a variety of clinical and managerial positions in acute and home care settings. Ms. Lovejoy has worked for the past 8 years with Visiting Nurses and Hospice of San Francisco. There, in addition to field work as an assessment nurse, she precepts, orients, and teaches documentation.

Making the Transition to Home Health Nursing

A Practical Guide

Denise Lovejoy, RN, MS

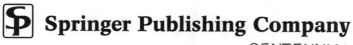

Springer Publishing Company

Springer Publishing Company, Inc.
536 Broadway
New York, NY 10012-3955

Cover design by Margaret Dunin
Acquisitions Editor: Ruth Chasek
Production Editor: Jeanne Libby

97 98 99 00 01 / 5 4 3 2 1

Library of Congress Cataloging-in-Publication Data

Printed in the United States of America

CONTENTS

PART III APPENDIXES

ACKNOWLEDGMENTS

Bringing an idea to life via a book is possible only with the support of many. Thanks to Pat Hess, Professor at San Francisco State University, who encouraged me to persevere and guided me through the several preparation steps. Norma Panina, Helen Wood, Carlos Miller, Robert Anderson, Kitty Wolfe, Fran Coperniak, Barbara Cymrot, Richard Wigen, and Mattie Attar, all professional colleagues, were very helpful in providing pieces of information necessary for accuracy. Their positive input was always welcomed. A special expression of gratitude to Susan Burlison, my husband Robert, and my son Mark, all of whom helped refine the presentation. Throughout the project, my family also greatly enhanced my appreciation of the beauty of the English language.

INTRODUCTION

Long gone are the days when home care was a refuge at the end of a nursing career. Once, tired of bedside nursing, nurses would change to public health, hoping for less stressful work. This very move indicated that they were one step closer to retirement. At least, that is how the change was perceived by nurses still doing "real nursing" in hospitals. Fortunately, both the image and the reality of home care have changed in recent decades. The Prospective Payment System was instituted by the federal government in response to escalating hospital costs, and also to reduce the many hospitalizations of an increasing elderly population. Patients' hospital stays became shorter. Home care demand, and work load, increased.

In the 1990s, the trend towards earlier discharges has accelerated. Efficiency in controlling cost is demanded by third-party payors. Hospitals are downsizing. Many nurses find themselves either changing careers or contemplating a change in specialty. Advances in medical technology have also facilitated caring for more patients in their homes. At the same time, to meet the challenge, many home health agencies have developed new specialty programs: wound, ostomy, perinatal-pediatry, and urology, for example. These have made home care more appealing to nurses looking for new opportunities to practice their expertise.

The terms "home care nursing" and "home health care nursing" are used interchangeably throughout the book, as well as the terms "speech-language pathology" and "speech therapy."

Changes are difficult, however. Nothing prepares nurses for the dramatic change from in-hospital service to the home setting, no matter how many years of experience they may have. I have been there. I struggled. I survived. Some of my co-workers did not. Learning autonomy of decision making, meeting multiple insurance requirements, and dealing with the formidable increase in paperwork are skills needed to function in the new environment. They must be learned.

This book is a guide to nurses entering the home health care field. Many nurses will have been practicing in hospitals and are now making the change. Others may have been out of the workforce for a while, or may be new graduates heading directly to this emerging opportunity. This book gives an overview of the specialty and shows how to make it from there to here. It identifies the good working habits necessary to acquire during the critical first months. The goal, then, is to facilitate the transition so that the rewards of the new specialty can be reaped sooner. A secondary goal is to present home care as an approachable alternative career for nurses considering a move.

The book is divided into three parts. Part I, *Understanding Home Care,* presents an overview of home care nursing, and as a point of reference, discusses the basic differences from hospital nursing. It also looks into the determining factors of a successful adaptation to the new specialty. Part II, *Home Care Nursing Practice,* covers the actual work of home care nursing, emphasizing the practical side. It particularly stresses important techniques of time management. The suggestions for the resolutions of difficulties, or their prevention, are a compilation of what I have learned, sometimes the hard way, both through experience and study of the literature. All suggestions are intended to be generic, and should not conflict with any agency's specific procedures. In a very practical way, this book complements existing home care manuals, to facilitate the application of their more clinical aspects to the actual home care nursing process. Part III, *Appendixes,* contains information pertinent to the daily activities of home care nurses.

Chapter 1 defines home health nursing and introduces its goals. Professional standards are the basis for home care nursing practice. They are reviewed and explained in this chapter. Major differences between hospital and home environments, and their effect on care delivery, are highlighted.

Chapter 2 presents the structure of home care, identifying types of agencies, regulatory bodies, and personnel. Sources of reimbursement are discussed, as well as the criteria that must be met when patients are admitted to the service.

Chapter 3 concentrates on important factors influencing the change to the home care specialty. Suggestions are made for an orientation program that can clarify, early on, some of the complexities of home care nursing, and provide a better understanding of the specialty's basics. The benchmarks of the transition are looked at, as well as the pitfalls. Perseverance brings rewards. Hints for a successful transition are given at the end of this chapter.

As the first section on *Home Care Nursing Practice,* Chapter 4 examines nursing work in the home. It is divided into three parts: before, during, and after the visit. The logistics of home visits, from referrals to visit completions, are explained. Suggestions are made throughout the chapters to assist with time constraints.

Chapter 5 looks at caseload management. Definition, responsibilities, resources, confidentiality, communications, time management, and quality assurance are all discussed. A short segment at the end explains how weekend and holiday work varies from work during the week. An overview of the organization, the personnel, and the selection of the patients to be visited completes the chapter.

People's homes are the determinants of the home care environment. Learning how best to operate within these milieus greatly facilitates the daily work. Chapter 6 introduces some characteristics of that environment. It also includes a section on safety and sexual harassment. Because travel time significantly influences nurses' productivity, the last section, "On the road," covers tips for safety, choices of routes, and parking. Information on timing of visits completes the chapter.

The six Appendixes include: (A) Medicare coverage of services; (B) abbreviations; (C) educational resources; (D) tools of the trade; (E) the car, presented as a vehicle, an office, and a classroom, with ways to minimize repairs and save fuel; things to do while driving so that time becomes learning time; and (F) occupational hazards and how to prevent them. The bibliography includes references used both in practice and in the preparation of this guide.

This book is a response to a newly developing need in the rapidly changing environment of caregiving. Written for practicing nurses making the transition from hospital to home care nursing, for nurses returning to the workforce, and new graduates, it can also be useful to student nurses in their community and home health clinical rotation.

The flexibility of home care nursing often comes as a surprise to nurses new to the specialty. It brings about a wonderful sense of freedom. The contrast with the strict schedule of institutional nursing gives almost a feeling of relief. It is one of the fringe benefits of this particular type of work. It is hoped that at the end of this book, you will have a better understanding of this growing specialty, and feel that its goals are not so out of reach after all.

PART I

UNDERSTANDING HOME CARE

Chapter 1

HOME CARE vs. HOSPITAL NURSING: A COMPARISON

A thorough understanding of the goal of home care is the starting point for a transition from institutional care. What is home care? In our constantly evolving health care system, there are several definitions currently used, each one based on the focus of its own organization. The National Association for Home Care, Medicare, the American Medical Association, and the American Hospital Association each provide us with their own. For nurses, the American Nurses Association (ANA) statement defines the responsibilities. A professional practice is based on standards. Home care nursing, as a specialty, has specific standards. Nurses making the move from hospital to home care must be aware of the additional accountability. This chapter covers both standards and the goals of home care nursing.

DEFINITION

"Home health nursing refers to the practice of nursing applied to a client with a health deficit in the client's place of residence" ANA (1992, p. 5). The focus of the practice is patients and their designated caregivers. Home care is multidisciplinary. Physical, occupational, and speech therapists; social workers; and home health aides all contribute to the well-being of the patients, and assist in carrying out the plan of care. Vendors and providers, who are the technical part of home care, dispense equipment and supplies. Nurses act as coordinators.

STANDARDS

The practice of home health nursing, as mentioned, is based on professional standards.

A standard is "a norm that expresses an agreed-upon level of excellence that has been developed to characterize, to measure, and to provide guidance for achieving excellence in practice" (ANA, 1986, p. 21). To the nurse learning the basics of a new specialty, the priority and importance of standards may not be obvious. However, agencies have integrated these standards throughout their policies and procedures. By striving to follow those guidelines, nurses new to home care will be one step closer to successfully making the change to the new field. The ANA standards are shown in Table 1.1.

GOALS

The practical, working goal of home care is to meet the health care needs of people within the limitations of cost reimbursement. However, "The goal of care" (nursing) "is to initiate, manage, and evaluate the resources needed to promote the client's optimal level of well-being" (ANA, 1992, p. 5). Home care provides a broad level of services more economically than do hospitals. Consequently, the nursing activities necessary to achieve the goal cannot ignore the cost constraints and limitations imposed by the various sources of reimbursement. Today's reality calls for creativity. Emphasis on restoration, maintenance, and prevention of potential problems is primary. Accomplishment of these goals is done by utilizing, through a three-stage process, the resources available to home care.

Initiating Resources

This stage commences with the admission interview/assessment process. Needs and outcomes are determined. The care plan is established. Suppliers for hospital beds and other equipment are selected. Other disciplines are integrated into the plan: Physical Therapy (PT), Occupational Therapy (OT), Speech Therapy (ST) to help rehabilitation; social workers, if emergency safety systems or home meals delivery, are needed; and home health aides to assist with personal care.

TABLE 1.1 The American Nurses Association Home Care Nursing Standards

Standard I. Organization of Home Health Services
All home health services are planned, organized, and directed by a master's-prepared professional nurse with experience in community health and administration.

Standard II. Theory
The nurse applies theoretical concepts as a basis for decisions in practice.

Standard III. Data Collection
The nurse continuously collects and records data that are comprehensive, accurate, and systematic.

Standard IV. Diagnosis
The nurse uses health assessment data to determine nursing diagnoses.

Standard V. Planning
The nurse develops care plans that establish goals. The care plan is based on nursing diagnoses and incorporates therapeutic, preventive, and rehabilitative nursing actions.

Standard VI. Intervention
The nurse, guided by the care plan, intervenes to provide comfort, to restore, improve, and promote health, to prevent complications and sequelae of illness, and to effect rehabilitation.

Standard VII. Evaluation
The nurse continually evaluates the client's and family's responses to interventions in order to determine progress toward goal attainment and to revise the data base, nursing diagnosis, and plan of care.

Standard VIII. Continuity of Care
The nurse is responsible for the client's appropriate and uninterrupted care along the health care continuum, and therefore uses discharge planning, case management, and coordination of community resources.

Standard IX. Interdisciplinary Collaboration
The nurse initiates and maintains a liaison relationship with all appropriate health care providers to assure that all efforts effectively complement one another.

Standard X. Professional Development
The nurse assumes responsibility for professional development and contributes to the professional growth of others.

Standard XI. Research
The nurse participates in research activities that contribute to the profession's continuing development of knowledge of home health care.

Standard XII. Ethics
The nurse uses the code for nurses established by the American Nurses Association as a guide for ethical decision making in practice.

Note. From *Standards of Home Health Nursing Practice* (pp. 5–19), 1986, Washington, DC: American Nurses Association. Copyright 1986 by the American Nurses Association. Reprinted with permission. Those seeking more details are advised to consult the standards and their interpretive statements.

Managing Resources

This is an ongoing process. Have workers in all the disciplines initiated their treatment in a timely manner, as the needs were determined on admission? Was the equipment delivered as ordered? Following up is a must for a plan to be effective. In home care, however, because nurses spend only a fraction of their day in the patients' homes, and do not enjoy constant contact with their co-workers, as in a hospital, the followup is more complicated.

Evaluating Resources

This is also an ongoing process. Are the needs of each individual patient being met with the resources determined in the original care plan? Are nursing consultations by specialists needed? Perhaps a patient is quite capable of taking care of himself and can be discharged after only two or three visits. A continuous assessment of the patient's response to treatment, and the methods used to meet the goals, is necessary to "promote the client's optimal level of well-being" (ANA, 1992, p. 5).

Home care nursing maximizes the efficacy of treatments and procedures performed or begun in hospitals. It is a bridge between subacute health situations and recovery. Reimbursement sources might change, environments of delivery might change, but nurses will always strive to meet the health care needs of their patients in a warm and sympathetic manner. This tradition remains.

DIFFERENCES

Nurses who have made the transition from hospital to home care have identified several difficulties. One study examined registered nurses in a bachelor's degree program during their clinical rotation in home care. The authors came to the same conclusion: the transfer of skills over to the new specialty was not easy (Ceslowitz & Loreti, 1991). The need to function as a generalist, the complexity of patient assessments, and documentation were particular problem areas. When nurses change specialties within an institution, the new skills seem to be learned faster than when transferring to home care. Why is this so? Home care is a specialty with a specific body of knowledge, not unlike oncology, orthopedics, or ostomy. The learning process involved should be the same. Evidence points to the fact that making the transition from institutional to home care is somehow more complex.

This chapter looks at the major differences between hospital and home care nursing. By comparing the two, we can see where the difficulties arise and thus understand their effect on care delivery.

The workers in both environments are the same. Beyond the distinctions of acute versus convalescent care, two major differences stand out between hospital and home care nursing. Home care requires greater *autonomy of decision making,* and also *increased responsibilities related to reimbursement.* Of course, nurses working in hospitals make decisions and prevent waste. They could not work as professionals without doing so. In home care, however, these two skills need to be further refined if one is to function effectively.

Autonomy of Decision Making

"Autonomous practice is built upon a body of expert knowledge. According to Mundinger, if the nurse has the knowledge and the skill to initiate and carry out actions, and to answer for the results, then the nurse is practicing autonomously" (Collins & Henderson, 1991, p. 23). By the time nurses complete training, they are in possession of theories and skills that allow them to make basic decisions about patient care. More knowledge and experience are necessary in order to function as a specialist. Home care, as a specialty, requires expert knowledge that can be learned, building on existing skills.

Fortunately, the home care environment provides what is necessary to promote self-sufficiency and autonomy of decision making. From the beginning, nurses making the move from hospitals can learn to bridge the gap and surmount the difficulties identified earlier.

In order to understand how the environment of care delivery can foster autonomy of decision making, let's compare the process of changing specialty in each of the two settings. First, within a hospital: For example, moving from a medical-surgical to an oncology unit; What environmental changes are encountered during the process?

Change within the Hospital Environment

Physical layout. Both units, the old and the new, are probably very similar: nursing station, well-lit patient rooms, medication and utility rooms, etc. A general orientation to the new floor plan can be done quickly by a preceptor, helping to familiarize the newcomers with their surroundings.

Without much delay, nurse and preceptor can start the morning routine together.

Daily basic nursing activities. Making out assignments, administering medications, assessing responses to treatments, and calculating intakes and outputs, to name only a few activities, do not change from unit to unit. In the example of a move from medical-surgical to oncology, however, in addition to the activities mentioned, there is a substantial increase in intravenous medications administration.

Teaching. Teaching, in hospitals, is an ongoing nursing activity. Due to a sharp decrease in length of stay, teaching must be done more quickly, no matter what specialty is involved. Visual approaches have to be utilized more often to reinforce instructions. Fortunately, the process started on one shift can be completed or reinforced on another. Information passed on to patients can be provided to families as well.

However, the logistics of coordinating patient/nurse/relatives' schedules are not always easy. Time is at a premium for all involved, and caregivers are not always available when nurses are ready to teach.

New body of knowledge. In the transition from medical-surgical to oncology nursing, the new body of knowledge inherent to the specialty includes learning about cancer development, nomenclature of malignant tumors, treatment modalities, and nursing management of patients undergoing chemotherapy. Also, learning how to deal with the multiplicity of vascular access devices becomes a very important part of the learning process.

Because of the many immunocompromised patients, and their special needs, the activity level of an oncology unit is intense. Nurses new to the specialty need to learn how to deal with the pace and the pressure.

Resources. Accessibility to resources in hospitals is excellent. Because of the hospital's high acuity, nurses are surrounded by invaluable and easily accessed resources. For any question that comes to mind, for any difficulty with a procedure, there is always a professional nearby who can come to the rescue immediately. Co-workers, house staff, and physicians are available and ready to assist. Cardiac arrest teams and intravenous (IV) teams are also at one's disposal. Pharmacists, nurse epidemiologists, and nutritionists are only a phone call or a few steps away.

By comparison, when nurses move from hospital to home care nursing, what differences are there in the changes encountered? More specifically, which changes foster autonomy of decision making?

Change from Hospital to Home Care

Physical layout. The physical environment of home care is neither familiar nor constant. From spectacular mansions to hotels and homeless shelters, home care nursing takes you where you are needed. Unsafe areas, requiring the protection of security escorts, are not uncommon. Thus, the variety in physical environment is the first dramatic change from hospital work, where the territory is familiar day after day.

Daily basic nursing activities. There are no set routines in home care. The main activity of the day is visits to patients' homes, each one presenting a different environment. Assessing health needs, monitoring effects and side effects of multiple medication regimens, changing dressings, and administering intravenous medications are some of the many activities filling nurses' days. Clinical skills necessary to perform those nursing activities are comparable to the ones needed in hospitals.

Much of the time, in home care, nurses have control over the scheduling of visits. Often, however, nurses must be flexible and accommodating; for example, when a patient is undergoing radiation or going to dialysis regularly. The same can be said of hospital work; procedures, tests, and treatments must be accommodated. The difference is that when patients return from the x-ray department, nurses do not have to drive 5 miles to go change the dressings. In addition, in home care practice, the need to accommodate access and schedule of other family caregivers is unique.

Another difference between hospital and home care is that the paperwork seems to increase tenfold. Documentation consumes a large portion of the home care nurse's day. Not only must progress notes be written after each visit, treatment plans have to be reevaluated every 62 days, rewritten, and sent to physicians.

Teaching. As far as teaching the patient is concerned, home care has a definite advantage over the hospital environment. Teaching in homes can be done over several visits. There is more time to assimilate into families and customize teaching. There are no other shifts to help share the instructions, however; nurses must follow through themselves, until completion.

As in scheduling, they must also take family dynamics in consideration. Are there in-home caregivers? When are they available? Are they receptive to teaching, or able to learn? These questions must be answered at the original assessment. But even with the best intention of helping humanity, nurses have to remember that they are on other people's territory. Being a guest means adapting to the environment, and working with people to attain goals.

New body of knowledge. Humphrey (1994) gives us an idea of the skills necessary for home care nurses to be effective in their new environment: "The ability to conduct a successful home visit is an art that requires skills of clinical practice, counseling, communication, and psychology as well as expertise in cultural, social, and community assessment" (p. 1). As degrees of expertise vary, so does clinical experience. Learning to adapt existing skills to the new, totally different environment is the challenge faced by nurses moving from hospital or other settings to home care nursing. Home care "is a practice area where one-to-one patient interaction still occurs. While practice is performed under a medical plan of treatment, it is the patients and home care professionals who provide the input for treatment plans and then consult the physician" (Brault, 1991, p. 8).

Resources. The lack of immediately available resources in home care situations is the single major factor promoting autonomy of decision making. Being on your own teaches you to trust your judgment, to draw from previous experience at the bedside, and apply that experience to the current problem. Dealing with a new difficulty successfully provides a base for handling the next one with confidence.

Who can be counted on as resources in home care and where can they be found? Co-workers, supervisors, and social workers are the most accessible. They can relate to the situations you are facing because they have experienced them themselves. They are only a beeper away! Pharmacists, nurse epidemiologists, and physicians can also be very helpful. The important subject of resources is looked at in more depth in Part Two, under *Caseload Management*.

Increased Responsibilities Related to Reimbursement

This is the second major difference between hospital and home care nursing. Reliance on home care has increased tremendously in recent years. Several studies have shown the cost-effectiveness of caring for patients in their homes, while a few others have challenged that benefit. Nevertheless, third-party payors have increased their utilization of home care, often using it as a substitute for hospitalization. Also, improvements in technology are permitting people to choose to be cared for in their own homes, where they do not lose control over their environment. Home visits by health professionals are reassuring for patients. Combined with the perceived cost-effectiveness for the insurers, home care benefits everyone. The individual home care nurse addresses this issue with every visit and every entry in the treatment plan. How does this compare to the hospital? Are nurses aware of reimbursement? Do budget constraints vary from one specialty to another?

Reimbursement within the Hospital

In 1982, the U.S. Department of Health and Human Services instituted the prospective reimbursement system for hospitals. This diagnostic-related groupings (DRGs) system of classification and reimbursement had the effect of decreasing patients' length of stay. Private insurance companies and state Medicaid followed suit and began restricting payments for hospitalizations. As a result, cost containment became the order of the day for hospitals nationwide, and that is true today more than ever.

How are hospital nurses affected by these new ways of reimbursement triggered by Medicare?

Generally, each nursing unit in a hospital is an individual cost center. In most hospitals, the budget is done once a year by the nurse-manager, working in cooperation with someone from the administrative organization. Staff nurses are made aware, at that time, of the "numbers" for the year, meaning how many staff members are allowed per shift, per unit, based on the number of patient days and the acuity from the previous year. Over the years, these "numbers" seldom seem to increase. However, the mix of employees—registered nurses, licensed vocational nurses, and aides—sometimes changes. This is a result of cuts in the general hospital budget, based in part on changes in reimbursement. Staff learns, early on, to adapt to budget limitations, and to reorganize their individual workloads to complete daily assignments in a timely manner. This is not always easy, but it is necessary.

Do budget constraints vary from one specialty to another? A move to our oncology example means, for nurses, simply adapting to the new unit's staffing pattern. Again, as a result of cost containment, these constraints are experienced in daily assignments. Without being aware of the specific reimbursement source for each individual patient, nurses on units are frequently reminded to conserve supplies, as part of cost containment in general. For example, linen is a major item. Patterns of replacing bedding are often adapted for linen conservation: for example, changing only draw sheets instead of entire bedding every day, or changing sheets every other or third day. Recently, gloves have also joined the list of items to conserve. Still, since the advent of universal precautions, staff members have recognized the importance of protecting themselves and their patients. A move to an oncology unit, as in our example, means the use of even more gloves and other supplies, due to the high acuity, and the increase in intravenous (IVs), syringes, and needles. Thus, the pattern changes somewhat with the character of the unit.

Reimbursement in Home Care

In home care, the issue is less of variable costs (supplies and labor) against fixed revenues (DRGs). Instead, it is an issue of ensuring reimbursement for a variable level of care determined, in large part, by the nurse's proficiency in documenting the need for that level of care.

Nurses moving to home care become quickly aware of how critical the reimbursement question is to every visit they make. Most likely, their preceptors have had to make several calls to insurers before setting out on the road to make "authorized" visits that day. Historically, there has always been a heavy emphasis on reimbursement in home care. However, as managed care is coming to the fore, fuelled by HMOs, cost containment is quickly becoming an issue for home care nurses. Each source of reimbursement has different allowances for services rendered. Nurses, as case managers, must then be aware of the funding source for each individual patient before they can either add another discipline or order supplies. The task is formidable, especially when a caseload constitutes 25–30 patients. "Cost-containment, not better care, is the third party payor's motivation for home care. The professional nurse must be alert to situations where home care is clearly not appropriate and assert the nurse's role as an advocate to see that the care indicated is provided" (Faherty, 1990, p. 13).

Most home care agencies are reimbursed by visits, the dollar amount varying from payor to payor. Nurses then are affected by shrinking reimbursement levels, so that their productivity (number of patients seen per week) must meet a sufficient volume for the agency to be viable and successful. This is in addition to closely monitoring each visit and all supplies ordered, following strict guidelines in order to ensure reimbursement.

What are the nursing goals for a given patient? How much time is allowed to accomplish these goals? The questions must be answered by home care nurses at the first visit, after the assessment. Because visits and supplies translate to dollars and cents, nurses enter the front line of reimbursement responsibility when moving from hospital or other settings to home care.

EFFECT ON CARE DELIVERY

How do the differences in the environment affect the delivery of nursing care?

Hospital

Hospital stays are now shorter. More tests and procedures are scheduled within shorter periods of time. Nurses must adjust quickly to the increased pace and crunch patient teaching into less and less time. Logically, decreased teaching time should foster creativity and encourage autonomy of decision making. However, this is not the case, because it is easier and faster to go with what you already know than to try new ways. Patients are also affected. Often, after overnight stays, when patients are still groggy from anesthesia, they have to memorize instructions. Remembering symptoms of infection or complications to report to their physicians is not easy, given their physical and emotional condition.

Patients and nurses alike feel the pressure of decreasing time between admissions and discharges. In general, there is less time for nurturing, or attempting to get to the roots of the problem that has, many times, caused the disease in the first place. The stability of a permanent, qualified staff can do wonders for patients' recovery. On the other hand, the uncertainty of job permanence, with health care institutions everywhere reorganizing and combining, can also have an effect on the nursing care delivery. Nervous energy prevails. In anticipation of major changes or layoffs, some nurses may resign. Registry nurses are often brought in to accommodate fluctuations in census. Fragmentation of care can be seen on many units. Nursing care plans are not always completed. Continuity somehow becomes a word of the past.

Home Care

Even when there are time constraints on the daily activities of home care nursing, the environment is kinder to nurses. The acuity is lower, even though early discharges from hospital produce sicker patients. More sophisticated technical skills are required. The plan of care, established at the first visit, can be implemented over a longer period of time. Consequently, as seen in the previous chapter, teaching can be spread out over several visits. Individual differences in the ability of patients and caregivers to grasp concepts and demonstrate skills can be accommodated.

Flexibility of schedule fosters creativity. Patients are under the care of physicians who have determined home health needs. Nurses decide how the goals are to be achieved, in each particular home situation, to fit the environment. It is very satisfying to see the improvement in health conditions resulting from the collaborative efforts of patients and health professionals.

Home care nursing can be compared to primary nursing. Continuity of care is achieved through case management. Occasionally, when caseloads become heavy, fragmentation of care can also be seen. However, it is fairly easy for nurses to know what to do at each visit, because nursing care plans are written at the initial visit, and problems are identified by order of importance.

Chapter 2

THE STRUCTURE OF HOME CARE

TYPES OF AGENCIES

Medicare is a federally funded insurance program for people 65 or older, people of any age with permanent kidney failure, and certain disabled persons under 65. With its passage in the 1960s came the proliferation of home health agencies. Diagnosis-related groupings (DRGs), federally mandated in the 1980s, decreased the patient's length of stay in the hospital, further encouraging the growth of agencies. Medicaid, a public assistance program administered by the states, followed, also decreasing payments for hospitalizations. These new pressures on reimbursement rates increased the need for, and the utilization of, home care alternatives. From 1967 to 1995, the number of Medicare Certified Health Agencies grew from only 1753 to 8747 (National Association for Home Care, 1995, p. 1).

These agencies, which provide nursing and other specialized services in homes rather than in the more expensive hospital settings, can be for-profit or not-for-profit. These financial designations apply to tax classification under the Internal Revenue Code. Terms like "government agency," "proprietary," or "church affiliated" refer, however, to ownership. Regardless of ownership or sponsoring source, most such agencies rely heavily on third-party payors such as Medicare, Medicaid, and insurance companies. In addition, all but government agencies also have a substantial number of private pay patients. Recently, out of economic necessity, the home care field has seen many mergers and changes that make the distinctions between types of agency even more confusing. The following discussion assumes the classifications commonly in use today (see Table 2.1).

Government Agencies

Government agencies provide home health services through the nursing divisions of state or local health departments. They are given their power through statutes enacted by legislation. "The organizational structure within the nursing divisions varies among agencies with some agencies opting to have their public health nurses include their home health clients within their overall public health caseload" (Harris, 1994, p. 16). Because of the proliferation of private agencies, and the high number of indigent patients, most public health services today are concentrating on disease prevention and communicable diseases. Environmental and maternal-child health are also major concerns. Funding comes from municipal, county, and state taxes.

Voluntary Agencies

Home health agencies that are not underwritten by state and local tax revenues but are financed primarily with nontax funds such as donations, endowments, and United Way contributions are called voluntary agencies. Visiting Nurse Associations are one example of this type. Voluntary agencies are governed by boards of directors composed of interested individuals who are part of the well-defined community they serve. The growth of private and institution-based home health agencies has eroded the referral sources of these agencies. Competition for patients has resulted in a decrease in their numbers in recent years.

Private Agencies

Most private agencies are for-profit, and are usually referred to as proprietary. As a result of consolidation, many proprietary agencies are now part of national chains and are administered through a corporate headquarters.

While the greater part of their revenues is generated through third-party payors, these agencies typically have a higher percentage of private pay patients. Acute and chronic home care nursing (versus only acute care for most Medicare-certified providers), private duty nursing, hospital staffing,

TABLE 2.1 Type of Agencies

Aspect of Agency	*Government*	*Voluntary*	*Proprietary*	*Institution Based*	*Hospice*	*Homemaker-Home Health Aide*
Governing body	Local government units (boards of supervisors, local board of health) by way of local health officer	Board of directors comprising members of service area and local community	Individual owner(s) or corporate headquarters (chain)	Sponsoring health organization's board of trustees	Board of directors comprising members of local community and service area (independent) or board of trustees of sponsoring health organization (institution based)	Individual owner(s) or corporate headquarters (chain)
Role of professional advisory committee	Functions in advisory capacity as defined in Medicare regulations	Functions in advisory capacity as defined in Medicare regulations	Functions in advisory capacity as defined in Medicare regulations	Functions in advisory capacity as defined in Medicare regulations	Closely knit team of professionals and volunteers provides services as well as consultation	Usually no professional advisory committee; comply with appropriate Medicare personnel standards if contracted by a Medicare-certified agency
Client case mix/services provided	Skilled home health clients; may have higher percentage of indigent; also, provides public health services such as maternal-child health, family planning, environmental health	Skilled home health clients of all ages, some screening activities such as health maintenance, other community health activities in senior centers, etc., services becoming more diverse.	Skilled home health clients of all ages; private duty services, hospital staffing services	Skilled home health clients of all ages; some custodial or private duty care	Terminally ill clients (usually with less than a 6-month life span prognosis), much involvement with significant others; bereavement services also provided; volunteers used for services provided	Skilled and unskilled (custodial) home health clients of all ages; personal care and housekeeping services provided
Revenue sources	Primarily from tax revenues, third party insurance payers (Medicare, medical assistance, Blue Cross/Blue Shield, etc.)	Donations (such as United Way), endowments, fund raising, third party insurance payers, private pay (usually on sliding fee basis)	Third party insurance payers, private pay	Third party insurance payers, private pay, donations, endowments, fund raising, usually in conjunction with sponsoring institution	Third party insurance payers (including Medicare hospice benefit), self-pay, donations, grants	Contract revenues from Medicare, certified home health agencies, private pay

Reprinted with permission, Harris, M.D., Handbook of Home Health Care Administration, 1994, (p. 19). Copyright 1994, Aspen Publishers, Inc.

and extended hours are some of the various services offered by private agencies.

Institution-Based Agencies

Hospitals may operate a home health agency as a separate department. The sponsoring organization's board of trustees or directors then govern the agency as well. The mission usually coincides with the hospital's. The inpatient population of the facility is the major source of referrals. Discharge coordinators, social workers, and liaison nurses become the case finders of potential home care patients. An advantage of institution-based agencies is the continuity of care. Patients generally appreciate it that the care being coordinated by persons familiar with the physicians and the institution.

Hospice

A hospice is defined by the National Hospice Organization (1984) as an agency for terminally ill patients in which "services are provided by a medically supervised interdisciplinary team of professionals and volunteers." The focus of the care is pain control and improvement of the quality of life. Holistic and interdisciplinary approaches are components of the hospice philosophy. While other home care agencies discontinue services when patients expire, hospice programs continue to support the families after the patient's demise.

The hospice admission criteria, as defined by Medicare, must include a diagnosis of a terminal illness, a prognosis of 6 months or less, a do-not-resuscitate order by the physician, and an informed consent from the patient.

Homemaker–Home Health Aide Agencies

The services provided by these agencies range from skilled to custodial. Home health aides concentrate on personal care and must be instructed and supervised regularly by a registered nurse as required by Medicare. Homemakers provide housekeeping services.

Agencies providing homemaker–home health aide services are typically private. Payment comes directly from the customers or from private insurances. The governing bodies can be individual owners or corporations. Many of these agencies are staffed by Medicare-certified home health aides who have passed competency evaluation tests. They contract out to home health agencies who can then bill Medicare for reimbursement.

Other Home Health Care Providers

High-technology nursing necessitates the use of specialized equipment. Durable medical equipment (DME) companies supply ventilators, parenteral and enteral nutrition supplies, pumps for continuous chemotherapy, etc., for home use. They fill the technical needs of home care, while the professional services come from one of the agencies described above.

REGULATORY BODIES

Medicare Conditions of Participation

Medicare reimbursement pays for as much as 59% of the care provided through home services. To receive Medicare benefits, home health agencies must follow the regulatory requirements called Conditions of Participation. These standards give direction to service providers and form the basis for evaluation of the quality of the services rendered. Each agency's policies and procedures incorporate these requirements, which affect the administrative as well as the field staff. By carefully following those policies and procedures, employees at all levels can help their agencies comply with the regulations, thus decreasing denials of visit reimbursements. Too many such denials can threaten an agency's viability.

The standards cover requirements pertinent to patients, to physicians, and to all disciplines and personnel. While administrators have the ultimate responsibility for meeting certification conditions, a team effort is necessary to achieve compliance in each department.

State Licensure

> Most states that have HHA (Home Health Agency) licensure laws make it a criminal offense for anyone to operate an HHA without a license. In many instances, however, the licensure requirement applies only to those HHAs that intend to participate in the Medicare or Medicaid program. An HHA that is treating only private insurance or private pay patients will not be required to be licensed (Harris, 1994, p. 86).

The operating standards set out by states are usually minimal, but must be followed at all times. Surveys by the state are done at regular intervals and determine eligibility for renewal. Some of the items looked at by the survey team are: skill levels of key personnel, compliance with applicable state and federal laws, and liability insurance coverage for all personnel. Unscheduled surveys may take place when a state receives complaints from patients. Investigation of possible noncompliance with licensure requirements usually follows such complaints. As part of state regulations, each patient must be informed of the State hotline number when admitted. (The State hotline is to the State Department of Health Services, Licensing and Certification Division. The purpose is to receive complaints or questions about local home health agencies.)

Accreditation

To participate in Medicare or Medicaid, home care agencies are required to have a state license. Accreditation, however, is not a requirement for such participation. Accreditation is a demonstration of a commitment to providing high quality care, and of having achieved higher standards of excellence. Accreditation may, however, be required for reimbursement by certain third-party payors. Meeting these more stringent standards demands a team effort from an agency's administrative staff, all personnel, and physicians; there is pride in achieving accreditation.

There are three nationally recognized organizations providing voluntary accreditation for home health agencies: The Joint Commission's Home Care Accreditation Program, The Community Health Accreditation Program (CHAP), and the National Home Caring Council.

JCAHO

The Joint Commission on Accreditation of Healthcare Organizations (JCAHO) is a private, not-for-profit organization dedicated to improving the quality of care provided to the public. JCAHO offers the Home Care Accreditation Program. The program survey covers patient-focused functions (ethics, rights and responsibilities; assessment; care; treatment; service; and education) and organizational functions (performance; leadership; management of environment of care, of human resources, and of information; control of infection).

A survey takes place at the request of the organization. The survey fee, which may present a substantial hurdle to many organizations, includes a fixed-base fee and an additional variable charge that is related to the type and volume of services, as well as how many offices may be included on the application provided by the applicant organization (Accreditation Manual for Home Care, 1995). The process includes interviews with administrators and field staff from different disciplines, home visits, and documentation review of patient charts, education materials, and governing body minutes. The patients to be visited are usually selected by the surveyors.

An agency is notified of the accreditation status after the review process. That status could be accreditation with commendation; accreditation; conditional; provisional; or denial. An organization has the right to appeal a decision of denial of accreditation.

CHAP

Another accreditation body for home health agencies is the Community Health Accreditation Program (CHAP), which is a subsidiary of the National League for Nursing (NLN). In 1992, CHAP was granted "deemed" status by the Department of Health and Human Services. "Deemed" status means that any home care agency that meets CHAP's accreditation standards will be considered to have met the federal government's conditions for participation in the Medicare and Medicaid programs.

Through an annual unannounced site visit, CHAP evaluates the quality of a home health agency. Home visits and telephone surveys are also done to assess patient satisfaction. An exit conference follows a visit, at which time the findings are discussed with the organization and recommendations are made.

National Home Caring Council

The third accreditation program is the National Home Caring Council, a division of the Foundation for Hospice and Homecare. The reality of agencies' limited financial resources is taken into consideration in the establishment of this organization's standards. Keeping in mind consumer safety and agency accountability, the standards reflect minimum requirements for operation. Recommendations usually follow a 2-day review visit, including interviews with a variety of individuals from the agency. Everyday activities are also compared with the agency's policies and procedures.

Home Health Care Organization

In order to compete in today's complex health environment, membership in a trade association is a must. The National Association for Home Care

(NAHC) fulfills that need as the nation's voice for home care. The association promotes trend-setting ideas, programs, and legislation on behalf of all those involved in home health care. Located in Washington, DC, NAHC remains in close contact with the White House, Congress, the Health Care Financing Administration (HCFA), the Veterans Administration (VA), and private enterprise, such as insurance companies. Among the many benefits NAHC offers its members are the latest statistics on home care, promotional items, videos, and brochures. It also publishes a journal, *Caring*, covering business and education issues of the home care industry.

With the goal of informing the public about ethical conduct for home health agencies and their employees, federal legislation requires that all agencies participating in the Medicare program have a patient bill of rights and responsibilities. This document, presented to all patients on admission to home care, must be fully explained. In addition to informing patients of both their rights and their responsibilities, the printed form helps make the home care relationship more concrete for both the health professional and the patient. Home care nursing is difficult to explain; this form gives an overview of certain actions that should occur in the home. These actions provide a suitable healing environment for the patients, and a safe one for the caregivers, nurses, and other health professionals. See the Homecare Bill of Rights as adopted by the National Association for Home Care, Table 2.2.

PERSONNEL

Administration, clinical management, and staff form the three major categories of personnel in most home care agencies. The number of employees in each category is determined by the type of agency, its size, and the number of programs being offered. With the many mergers reshaping the health industry today, the responsibilities of administrators and managers are changing constantly, in an effort to adapt. Here follow the types of positions seen typically in home health agencies:

Administration

The administrative or executive functions are those common to any operation, whether for-profit or not. They would include the executive, operational, and finance heads, although some agency executives may serve in more than one role. Examples are Executive Director or Chief Executive

TABLE 2.2 Home Care Bill of Rights

Home care clients have a right to be notified in writing of their rights and obligations before treatment begins and to exercise those rights. The client's family or guardian may exercise the client's rights when the client has been judged incompetent. Home care providers have an obligation to protect and promote the rights of their clients, including the following rights.

Clients and Providers Have a Right to Dignity and Respect

Home care clients and their formal caregivers have a right to not be discriminated against based on race, color, religion, national origin, age, sex, or handicap. Furthermore, clients and caregivers have a right to mutual respect and dignity, including respect for property. Caregivers are prohibited from accepting personal gifts and borrowing from clients.

Clients have the right:

- to have relationships with home care providers that are based on honesty and ethical standards of conduct;
- to be informed of the procedure they can follow to lodge complaints with the home care provider about the care that is, or fails to be, furnished, and regarding a lack of respect for property. (To lodge complaints with us call ______________);
- to know about the disposition of such complaints;
- to voice their grievances without fear of discrimination or reprisal for having done so; and to be advised of the telephone number and hours of operation of the state's home health "hot line," which receives complaints or questions about local home care agencies. The hours are __________ and the number is ______________.

Decision Making

Clients have the right:

- to be notified in advance about the care that is to be furnished, the types (disciplines) of the caregivers who will furnish the care, and the frequency of the visits that are proposed to be furnished;
- to be advised of any change in the plan of care before the change is made;
- to participate in the planning of the care and in planning changes in the care, and to be advised that they have the right to do so;
- to be informed in writing of rights under state law to make decisions concerning medical care including the right to accept or refuse treatment and the right to formulate advance directives;
- to be informed in writing of policies and procedures for implementing advance directives including any limitations if the provider cannot implement an advance directive on the basis of conscience;

(continued)

TABLE 2.2 ***(continued)***

- to have health care providers comply with advance directives in accordance with state law requirements;
- to receive care without condition on, or discrimination based on, the execution of advance directives; and
- to refuse services without fear of reprisal or discrimination.

The home care provider or the client's physician may be forced to refer the client to another source of care if the client's refusal to comply with the plan of care threatens to compromise the provider's commitment to quality care.

Privacy

Clients have the right:

- to confidentiality of the medical record as well as information about their health, social, and financial circumstances and about what takes place in the home; and
- to expect the home care provider to release information only as required by law or authorized by the client and to be informed of procedures for disclosure.

Financial Information

Clients have the right:

- to be informed of the extent to which payment may be expected from Medicare, Medicaid, or any other payor known to the home care provider;
- to be informed of the charges that will not be covered by Medicare;
- to be informed of the charges for which the client may be liable;
- to receive this information, orally and in writing, before care is initiated and within 30 calendar days of the date the home care provider becomes aware of any changes; and
- to have access, upon request, to all bills for service the client has received regardless of whether the bills are paid out-of-pocket or by another party.

Quality of Care

Clients have the right:

- to receive care of the highest quality;
- in general, to be admitted by a home provider only if it has the resources needed to provide the care safely and at the required level of intensity, as determined by a professional assessment; a provider with less than optimal resources may nevertheless admit the client if a more appropriate provider is not available, but only after fully informing the client of the provider's limitations and the lack of suitable alternative arrangements; and
- to be told what to do in the case of an emergency.

(continued)

TABLE 2.2 *(continued)*

The home care provider shall assure that:

- all medically related home care is provided in accordance with physicians' orders and that a plan of care specifies the services and their frequency and duration; and
- all medically related personal care is provided by an appropriately trained home care aide who is supervised by a nurse or other qualified home care professional.

Client Responsibility

Clients have the responsibility:

- to notify the provider of changes in their condition (e.g., hospitalization, changes in the plan of care, symptoms to be reported);
- to follow the plan of care,
- to notify the provider if the visit schedule needs to be changed;
- to inform providers of the existence of, and any changes made to, advance directives;
- to advise the provider of any problems or dissatisfaction with the services provided;
- to provide a safe environment for care to be provided; and
- to carry out mutually agreed responsibilities.

To satisfy the Medicare certification requirements, the Health Care Financing Administration requires that agencies:

1. Give a copy of the Bill of Rights to each patient in the course of the admission process.
2. Explain the Bill of Rights to the patient and document that this has been done.

To minimize confusion, NAHC recommends that agencies have clients sign one form that shows that the client acknowledges all of the agency's policies and procedures (e.g., release of medical information, billing procedures).

Note. From Home Care Bill of Rights by National Association for Home Care, 1993. Washington, DC: Author. Copyright 1993 by NAHC. Reprinted with permission. Not for further reproduction.

Officer (CEO); Assistant Director or Chief Operating Officer (COO); and Finance Director or Chief Financial Officer (CFO).

For agencies operating under Medicare Conditions of Participation, professional standards and credential requirements for administrators are found in the Conditions. Each state's guidelines might also contain administrative requirements.

Clinical Management

Director of Clinical Services

Clinical Management may be headed by the COO, if that person has a professional background. Otherwise, the top management role is generally that of the Director of Clinical Services. Other supervisors report to this top professional. Maintaining professional standards of patient care, and compliance with the various regulatory requirements, is the main responsibility of this position. In larger agencies, that person also oversees the specialty programs.

Supervisors

The organization of a home care office reflects the districts of the city it serves. The divisions are determined by each agency, usually to accommodate travel time for field staff. They can be based on zip codes, density of population, or patient acuity. There are usually as many teams or units in an office as there are divisions in a territory. Each team is headed by a supervisor who coordinates the care provided by the nursing staff. Often, a charge nurse on each team assists the supervisor with patient scheduling and the daily operations of that particular team.

Other programs, such as managed care, hospice, AIDS, and IVs can produce even more sections in an agency. Supervisors may be in charge of a single team or may cover two or three, depending again on the size and nature of the agency.

An intake or registration supervisor oversees a group of nurses and clerical staff who process referrals. In institution-based agencies, hospital liaison nurses work closely with physicians and discharge coordinators. They handle the discharges of patients referred to home care services. They are the go-betweens who link acute care institutions and the registration office of an agency.

Home health aides provide intermittent care to patients. A supervisor is in charge of scheduling for all home health aides, and manages personnel-related issues.

Staff

Nurses

In most agencies, registered nurses (RNs) comprise the largest number of personnel for the delivery of care at home. Their background may vary from associate degree to diploma, to bachelor's, and to master's-prepared. American Nurses Association (ANA) recommends the baccalaureate level for meeting the high standards of home health nursing practice. We find various positions operating on the nursing staff. For example, in some agencies assessment nurses make the initial home visit, determine needs, and hand the patients over to other RNs for case management. Case managers are responsible for coordinating the care of a group of patients. Caseload management is covered in detail in Chapter 5.

Nurse Specialists

Diabetic, enterostomal, psychiatric, pediatric, maternal-child, and pulmonary specialists, among others, provide direct patient care, in addition to doing consultations for other staff members. Inservice education is also part of their responsibility. Specialists in quality improvement and education are two other positions seen in agencies; these roles are often combined.

Licensed Vocational Nurses, Licensed Practical Nurses

Licensed Vocational Nurses (LVNs), called also Licensed Practical Nurses (LPNs) in some states, provide direct patient care under the supervision of an RN. "The specific skills that an LPN can deliver to a home care client and the type of reimbursement are governed by the state nurse practice acts, state licensure laws for home health agencies, and the policies of various reimbursement sources, and the policies of the home health agency" (Humphrey & Milone-Nuzzo, 1996, p. 7).

Physical, Occupational, Speech Therapists

Home rehabilitation is the territory of Physical Therapists (PTs), Physical Therapist Assistants (PTAs), Occupational Therapists (OTs), and Speech Therapists (STs). Safety in homes and use of appropriate equipment is the PT's and OT's main concern. Speech therapists concentrate on swallowing and speech difficulties. In order for the services to be reimbursed by Medicare, treatment plans must reflect patient functional limitations.

Respiratory Therapists

For patients on ventilators, a few agencies work on a contractual basis with Respiratory Therapists (RTs) if they do not have pulmonary specialist nurses on their staff. Treatments, handling of equipment, and inservice to the staff are some of their duties.

Social Workers

Among their many functions, Medical Social Workers (MSWs) identify patient and family psychosocial needs and handle referrals to community resources. They are tremendous resources for nurses and other health professionals. See Chapter 5, *Resources*, for more details about indications for referrals.

Nutritionists

Nutritionists provide consultations, usually on a contractual basis. Special diets, caloric intake in patients with tube feedings, and severe weight loss are some of the problems they handle. The direct service of a nutritionist is not a reimbursable home care service.

Home Health Aides

Home Health Aides (HHAs) provide hands-on personal care in the patients' homes, on a part-time or intermittent basis. Other activities include changing bed linens, assistance with transfers, and feeding. The purpose of a Home Health Aide visit must be to perform a health-related service to be reimbursable even though some incidental services may be performed during the visit (Medicare Health Insurance Manual (HIM–11)). The three aspects of the care provided are "personal care, extension of skilled nursing services, and extension of rehabilitation services" (Gilbert, 1992, p. 13). As part of the health home care team, the goals of Home Health Aides are to assist patients in their recovery and to provide a safer and more sanitary environment in which healing can take place.

Homemakers

Homemakers assist with household tasks such as preparing meals, doing the laundry, errands, and grocery shopping. Heavy housework is usually not part of their duties, nor is personal care as provided by HHAs.

Depending on the type of agency, HHAs, Personal Care Aides (PCAs), or Homemakers may be utilized. While some of their functions overlap, homemakers cannot perform the personal care provided by Home Health Aides. Certified agencies use HHAs; agencies that are licensed only, use HHAs, PCAs, and Homemakers.

Office Staff

Agency office staff can be divided into two groups: the business staff, and the support staff. The business staff deals with the financial aspect of the business, such as reimbursement, billing, and payroll. The support staff assists supervisors and other health professionals in handling the everyday activities pertinent to patients. This latter group might include unit coordinators, intermediate clerks, file clerks, and medical word processors, depending on the size of an agency. Each category of worker has a distinct job description, but they all work together in close cooperation. Often, some of the duties overlap.

Office personnel play a very important part in facilitating the work of the professional staff. Many questions need to be answered when beginning a new job. While many are pertinent to home care and can only be answered by other health workers, many address direction of paper flow or data retrieval from the computer. The office workers are familiar with all the forms; they handle them every day. They can direct you to the correct resources, if they don't have the answers themselves. Unlike the field staff who are in and out, the support staff are in place all day. They create the atmosphere of the office. In addition to their regular tasks, they remind you of deadlines, so you can meet some of your commitments. They also acknowledge birthdays and special events. How do they put up with the constant comings and goings of the field staff, politely answer the patients calling with their problems, direct all those calls, and still keep their sense of humor? Whatever their secret, it is one more reason to treat them with respect.

Escorts

Because of the high crime areas required to be covered by some agencies, security escort services may be used. The service is usually on a contractual basis and is not reimbursable.

REIMBURSEMENT

Who pays for the care you provide? In home health, the ability to deliver care is a function of the ability to be paid for the delivery of that care. Reimbursement sources influence how, by whom, and for how long home services will be rendered. Health professionals do, however, have control over the quality of the care they provide. Most important, by following certain guidelines, reimbursement can be maximized without compromising quality.

What are the main sources of reimbursement for home care agencies (see Table 2.3)? What are those guidelines? Where do you find them?

Medicare

Medicare (Title 18, Social Security Act, 1966) is the principal reimbursement source in home care. The program is administered by a branch of the federal Health and Human Services Department called the Health Care Financing Administration (HCFA). This department establishes guidelines and regulations which affect how nursing is paid for for Medicare patients. The document where these regulations can be found is called the *Medicare Health Insurance Manual–11,* otherwise referred to as the HIM–11 by all enlightened home care health professionals. Guidelines cover nursing, therapy, social services, and Home Health Aides. During orientation, field staff is taught the Medicare requirements and how they apply, both to admission to home care services and to the documentation of the care provided.

Various insurance companies act as fiscal intermediaries (FIs) for Medicare. "The FIs are responsible for determining whether services provided meet the federal guidelines. If services have not met these guidelines, the FI denies payment. This denial of payment is critical to Medicare agencies because it comes after the services have been provided" (Gabe & Gill-Forney, 1993, p. 31).

According to the HCFA requirements, five criteria must be met when a patient is admitted for home care services. These criteria are covered under four guidelines, the last two both being stated under Guideline 4. Here they are, as listed in the Medicare Health Insurance Manual (HIM–11):

1. Reasonable and Necessary Services (203.1)

Is there a medical need? Possibly there is an exacerbation of an existing condition. Both treatment plan and nursing care plan must reflect the patient's need. The home setting must be appropriate for these needs to be met.

TABLE 2.3 Sources of Payment for Home Care 1992 and 1994

Source of Payment	1992 All Home Care[1]	1994 Home Health Care (Current Clients)[2]
Total	**100.0%**	**100.0%**
Medicare	37.8	60.0
Medicaid	24.7	14.4
Private insurance	5.5	8.4
Out-of-pocket	31.4	3.1
Other & unknown	0.6	14.1

Sources: [1]NMES 1987 data and Lewin-VHI analysis for 1992. Based on total spending for home care.
[2]NCHS; unpublished data from the 1994 National Home and Hospice Care Survey. Based on source that paid the greatest amount during the last recorded billing period.
Note. From *Basic Statistics About Home Care* (p. 6), by National Association for Home Care (1996). Washington, DC: Author. Copyright by the National Association for Home Care. Reprinted by permission.

2. *Confined to the Home (204.1)*

The patient is homebound if he/she experiences:

A normal inability to leave home;
A considerable and taxing effort to leave; and
Absences from home are infrequent, of short duration, or to receive medical care.

Homebound eligibility is not affected by frequent absences from the home WHEN the reason to leave is to receive medical care.

Homebound criteria may be met when the beneficiary attends adult day care when the purpose is attributable to the patient receiving medical care.

3. *Services are Provided Under a Plan of Care Established and Approved by a Physician (204.2)*

A medical treatment plan indicating which services need to be provided must be determined by a physician, with the assistance of a home care nurse, or therapist. The content of the plan of care must be very specific, according to the guidelines. It needs to include: diagnoses, patient's mental status, types of services, supplies and equipment ordered, visit frequencies, prognosis, rehabilitation potential, functional limitations, activities permitted, diet, medications including over-the-counter medicines, safety measures, discharge plans, . . . "and any additional items the home health agency or physician choose to include."

4. Needs Skilled Nursing Care on an Intermittent Basis, or Physical Therapy or Speech Therapy or Has a Continued Need for Occupational Therapy (204.4)

This guideline covers two important criteria: skilled services and intermittent care. Could a nonmedical person provide these services? In determining if a service is considered skilled, HIM–11 recommends considering the inherent complexity of the service; the condition of the patient; and accepted standards of medical and nursing practice. Is the care intermittent? Frequency of home visits is determined by needs, and usually means several times a week for the duration of a treatment plan. If necessary, daily visits can be made for a short period of time. The treatment plan must be reviewed periodically, and frequency adjusted if appropriate. As for other criteria, interventions and outcomes must be clearly documented, on an ongoing basis.

Deciphering Medicare terminology and its application is not easy. Copies of the HIM–11 will be found in each agency. In addition there are, on the market, several good reference books for more information on the application of the guidelines; a few give examples for each criterion. See also Appendix A.

Medicaid

Medicaid (Title 19, Social Security Act) is another source of reimbursement. It is a federally aided, state-operated and state-administered program providing medical benefits for low-income persons. Each state determines program eligibility, benefits covered, and rates of payment for the providers. Clinical guidelines for eligibility follow those of the Medicare program. According to HCFA, Division of Medicaid Statistics, in 1994, of the $108 billion spent in Medicaid benefit payments, more than half went for hospital and skilled nursing facility services. Home health services comprised about 6.5% of the payments (National Association for Home Care, 1995, p. 4).

Private Insurance

Three major types of organizations provide health care reimbursement in the private sector: indemnity insurance companies that pay a percentage of billed charges, nonprofit Blue Cross and Blue Shield, and HMOs (MacLaren, 1994, p. 10). Health maintenance organizations (HMOs) offer comprehensive prepaid health care; they fall under the generic term of "managed care." The services covered vary by payor, but again, the documentation and clinical guidelines follow Medicare standards. Pre-authorization of visits is often required.

Indigent Care

Some medically indigent patients are referred to nonprofit agencies to be seen at no charge. Guidelines regarding admission to service, visits, and supplies are usually found in each agency's policies and procedures manual.

Chapter 3

ADAPTING TO THE HOME CARE SETTING

DETERMINING FACTORS FOR SUCCESS

Elements of excitement and of surprise often accompany change. Discovering a new world within nursing is certainly cause for enthusiasm. But the new territory may also trigger some measure of fear. The fear may be of not knowing how to apply the old skills to the new environment, or of not learning the new skills quickly enough to feel comfortable again.

Four factors influence a successful transition, help dissipate those fears, and keep enthusiasm alive: the preceptor, orientation, the supervisor, and the support group. This chapter looks at each factor, and makes suggestions to ease some of the difficulties. Much information is passed on during the first weeks of orientation. In order to retain much of that instruction, the learner must have a context to put it in or familiar situations to relate to. Therefore, it is important to start with the familiar, at the beginning of orientation, to build on existing knowledge before moving on to the new.

Preceptor

Orientation in the familiar hospital setting revolves around the ward or unit. Because of the decentralized activity in home health nursing, which takes place in various homes, the role of the preceptor in home care assumes even greater significance. A specific preceptor is usually assigned for the entire orientation period, and serves as a resource for the next 2–3 months thereafter. The quality of the precepting influences greatly the outcome of the orientation, and of the change to the new environment. Those selected as preceptors should be experienced, skilled nurses, preferably those who have retained their enthusiasm and sense of humor after a few years in the field. The ability to look at situations for what they are, without making judgements, comes with experience and maturity.

Newcomers need to be exposed to nurses who are skilled and compassionate, but also lighthearted. That kind of positive attitude will go a long way toward alleviating initial anxiety, thereby creating a better learning environment.

The role of a preceptor is to serve as the primary resource both during initial orientation and the first few months that follow. Preceptors' responsibilities are to identify the strengths and weaknesses of the new employee, meet the learning needs, and introduce the daily routine.

Several of the subjects otherwise incorporated in the orientation can be covered by the preceptor instead. Topics suitable for this alternative include:

1. Organization of a caseload: daily activities, and review of the treatment plan every 62 days (recertification); application of nursing process; contact with payor sources.
2. Time management.
3. Paper flow.

The preceptor should also stress the importance of:

1. Following up with patients' orders, lab reports, or other problems. Being responsible and accountable is the essence of home care.
2. Accessing resources immediately when in doubt about a course of action in a home.
3. Participating in staff meetings. Staff meetings give staff members the opportunity to get to know others, their strengths, and their availability as resources. In addition, case presentation is a great way to learn how to handle difficult situations in homes.
4. Discussing stressful experiences during a visit with another experienced nurse or supervisor, if the preceptor is not available. This helps put situations into perspective and can release some of the tension associated with the incident. An effective preceptor helps build a novice's confidence. During a transition process, the assurance that you are valued and needed as a skilled professional makes adapting to the environment much easier.

Orientation

The logistics of home care orientation programs are complicated. The various specialists invited to give presentations must also accommodate their own caseloads. Simply compiling a schedule of classes can become an ordeal; presenters come and go, not easily seen or met, because of the decentralized nature of the specialty.

Coordinating classes with home visits also presents difficulties not found in the hospital. Here, the patient might not be available when preceptor and nurse are otherwise free to visit. Considering their challenges, orientation coordinators deserve a lot of respect for their perseverance.

Orientation programs abound, each one with a different approach. Table 3.1 is an extract from section 2 of the Joint Commission on Accreditation of Healthcare Organizations (JCAHO), "Management of Human Resources." It provides a core list of subjects to be addressed during orientation.

Employees new to home care come from diverse educational backgrounds and work environments. In addition to those listed above, here are a few suggestions of topics to be added to facilitate the transition of new employees and give insight into the changes ahead:

- home care definition and goals;
- major differences between hospital and home care nursing;
- mission statement of the agency;
- nursing process;
- resources;
- *Homecare Bill of Rights;*
- communication;
- legal and ethical issues;
- caseload management;
- supervision;
- and safety in the field.

Special emphasis should be given to the subjects of reimbursement and documentation. Learning, at the beginning, how closely these two are linked can greatly influence the new staff member's way of looking at home care nursing.

The organization of such a substantial list of topics will vary, of course, from agency to agency. By knowing what is coming, however, the new team members can begin to form a context for learning. Remember, nurses will be far more "on their own" than in former hospital days, or wherever their previous care settings were. The sooner habits of independence and self-responsibility are formed, the smoother their transition will be.

TABLE 3.1 JCAHO Orientation Topics

- Types of care or service to be delivered in the patient's environment.
- Equipment management, including safe and appropriate use of equipment as applicable to care or service provided:
    - Individuals responsible for maintaining equipment demonstrate knowledge and competence in appropriate maintenance procedures for all equipment.
    - When required by the manufacturer, individuals responsible for preventive maintenance successfully complete the manufacturer's training program or another training program with equivalent content.
- Home safety issues, including bathroom, fire, environmental, and electrical safety.
- The storage, handling, and access to supplies, medical gases, and drugs appropriate to the care/services provided.
- The identification, handling, and disposal of hazardous or infectious materials and wastes in a safe and sanitary manner and in accordance with law and regulation.
- Infection control, including: personal hygiene, precautions to be taken, aseptic procedures, communicable infections and appropriate cleaning, disinfection, and/or sterilization of equipment and supplies.
- Confidentiality of patient information.
- Appropriate policies and procedures.
- Community resources as applicable to the care or service provided.
- Guidelines for appropriate referrals, including timeliness.
- Appropriate action in unsafe situations.
- Any specific tests to be performed by the staff.
- As appropriate, the organization's policies and procedures regarding advance directives.
- Organizational policies and procedures regarding death and dying.
- Screening for abuse and neglect, appropriate to the staff member's role and responsibility.
- Emergency preparedness.
- Any other patient care responsibilities.
- Gathering of information by staff regarding the care or service provided by other members of the staff, in order to better coordinate and appropriately refer the patient.

Note. From Accreditation manual for home care, Vol. 2 (1995). Oakbrook Terrace, IL: Joint Commission on Accreditation of Healthcare Organizations. Copyright 1995 by JCAHO. Reprinted with permission.

General Considerations Regarding Orientation Programs

The following are based on my own early difficulties, my subsequent home care experience, and, finally, my review of several orientation manuals.

1. Ideally, the program should have new orientees witness a home visit on the first or second day of orientation. If this can be a new admission, so much the better. This visit does not necessarily have to be with the preceptor. The idea is to experience home care, and see how nursing skills are applied in the new environment.
2. Teaching should be more from the familiar to the unfamiliar. Discharge forms, referrals, and the nursing process are known to hospital nurses and therefore are a good place to start.
3. Repetition is useful and necessary; there is much new material to be learned. Along with new material, each class session should reinforce the most important points from previous classes.
4. Introducing the paper flow is time-consuming; have the preceptor do so while teaching the daily routine. The orientee will remember forms more easily while actually using them.
5. Stress the importance of policy and procedure manuals for reference. In addition, recommend the two or three basic home care books most consistent with the particular agency's way of doing things.
6. Handouts are useful references. Here are some that are especially pertinent to day to day practice: *Homecare Bill of Rights;* copy of *Medicare Health Insurance Manual–11* (HIM–11); do's and don'ts of documentation; criteria for admissions, specialty consultations, PT, OT, ST, MSW, HHA; and lists of: employees' beepers and voice mail numbers; hospitals; ambulances; ambulatory services such as portable x-rays and EKGs; pharmacies that deliver; acceptable abbreviations; unsafe areas necessitating security escorts.
7. The entire orientation program could be divided into 2 parts, 2 weeks at the beginning and another week a month later. The continuation of the orientation process could include new subjects, and the reintroduction of others discussed in the first 2 weeks.

After having been exposed to home care work through joint visits with the preceptor, relating to the new information provided should be easier. At that time it would be appropriate to take up: organization of home health care system; administrative structure of agency; caseload management; supervision; documentation and reimbursement; quality assurance; noncompliance; recommendations of home health care and nursing clinical magazines; case presentations. Custom-designing a home care orientation program to fit every nurse's background is clearly impossible. The material to be covered is extensive and very different from other specialties. Whatever their background or level of expertise, nurses need to hear the information several times. Reintroducing some of the subjects presented during the first weeks is necessary to reinforce the important concepts. After having been in the field for a month or so, orientees will more readily understand the material presented and also be able to correct any prior misconceptions.

Again, each agency will offer a different orientation. To the extent necessary, these guidelines will also permit each nurse to seek out for themselves any important items not otherwise covered.

Supervisor

As compared to the nurses in the field, the supervisor's role shows some similarities between hospital setting and home care agency. In both we find: quality improvement, infection control, education, documentation, incident reports, evaluations, to name only a few. Some of the familiar hospital regulatory agencies regulate home care agencies as well. In addition to ensuring quality care in the home, rules have to be followed for accreditation and reimbursement. The supervisor's primary function is to maintain those standards, while orienting new employees to the necessary rules and regulations, and keeping everyone abreast of changes. Next, the supervisor must train staff members not only to work independently, while providing safe and competent care, but to grow in the process. This last function, a formidable task in itself is, however, the major reward of supervisory work in home care.

During orientation, supervisors can make newcomers feel more confident by providing professional guidance. A weekly meeting between supervisor, orientee, and preceptor, to review the progress made and reevaluate the clinical needs, is recommended. After the formal orientation is completed, meeting every other week is sufficient, unless there are some major difficulties with adaptation. What subjects should be on the agenda? Here are a few suggestions.

1. The past week(s) in review.
2. Positive experience in a home, reinforcing existing clinical knowledge of the orientee.
3. Any specific difficulties encountered in adapting to the new environment.

4. Ethical issues, including both the determination and limit of agency's responsibility.
5. Problematic patient behavior.
6. Clinical skills to concentrate on for the coming week(s).

Time being at a premium for all concerned, all these subjects need not be presented at each meeting. However, the nurse should be given the opportunity, at each conference, to report on a particular event or the handling of a situation that generated a good feeling about the new nursing field.

Supervisors need to emphasize to new orientees the importance of learning new clinical skills (for example, IV therapy, blood draw, use of pumps, glucometers). By doing so, both the individual nurse and the agency become more flexible and able to serve a broader group of patients. This is an advantage neither party can ignore in view of the tremendous changes taking place in health care today. In addition, it helps make the daily work much more interesting, which is the principal reason nurses are going to really enjoy their new career in home care.

Support Group

As orientation in a new specialty progresses within a hospital, nurses immediately tend to feel part of the team. The opposite must be guarded against when changing to home care. The transition from close work with a group of nurses to solo practice in the field can be a very isolating experience, despite all the best efforts of instructors, preceptor, and staff. So many changes take place in such a short time. In addition, the Medicare or agency regulations orientees are struggling to learn are subject to frequent revisions. Such is the current state of health care, with agencies working constantly to keep up. All these concerns can increase the stress level, calling for more peer support. Ideally, the new agency will provide for a support group, starting after orientation and continuing for the next 5 to 6 months. If no support group exists, nurses would be well advised to informally create their own.

The group's goals would be decreased stress, increased job satisfaction, and to assist in personal and professional development. Patients are sure to benefit from having nurses who are more comfortable and confident in their new role. By comparing notes with experienced nurses, newcomers soon discover that many of the difficulties they encounter do not necessarily stem from their own inexperience; they are, indeed, shared by many other staff members. For example, such problems as patients' noncompliance with the treatment plans are never-ending. Health care professionals' approaches differ; so do people's receptivity to new methods. It is not uncommon for nurses to think that inexperience prevents their teaching from being effective. Even if the group provides few "solutions" to such problems, the understanding and perspective offered can dramatically facilitate the new nurse's transition.

What would the "ideal" support group look like? Here are a few suggestions:

1. A specialist should lead the group. A psychiatric nurse, a clinical nurse specialist (CNS) with experience in leading support groups, a psychologist or a psychiatrist, are all good choices.
2. While staff members should be encouraged to attend meetings, attendance should not be mandatory.
3. The group should include a mix of both new and experienced registered nurses. All other health professionals should be encouraged to participate.
4. Under agency sponsorship, the program will be ongoing and the rules established. For more informal efforts, such issues should be addressed at the first meeting: frequency of meetings, commitment of members, confidentiality issue, and termination of individual membership.

An effective support group should make members feel better about themselves, and more at ease in the working environment. It should be a positive experience, not a drudgery or an obligation. One great benefit is that it allows the home health care nurse to see co-workers in a new light and learn to trust them as resources. Making a successful transition to home care calls for assistance from many people. Nurses can best find that kind of help from peers in a support group, where the atmosphere is more relaxed.

BENCHMARKS OF TRANSITION

A benchmark is a point of reference from which measurements can be made. When learning the specialty of home care, these reference points, acknowledged by experienced nurses, are to be found at about the 3rd and 6th months. In the context of a transition, progress toward both autonomy of decision making and increased responsibilities related to reimbursement is most noticeable at those particular times. By then, the orientation period and the actual work in the field will have answered many nurses' questions about their new specialty. These experiences will also have triggered many more questions that steady communication with, and assistance from, peers will eventually answer.

After about 3 months in the new specialty, nurses have a general sense of home care and how personal efforts contribute to the patients' recovery. The routine of the day and the paper flow have become familiar, if not yet under total control. Able and willing resources have been identified and consulted numerous times. Needed clinical skills have surfaced. Many decisions regarding treatment applications in homes have been taken independently, to the orientee's own satisfaction as well as that of the preceptor. After calling third-party payors several times, awareness of cost containment has already increased tremendously.

With this much progress made, what remains? Time is still the enemy. The positive feeling of being able to apply old skills in the new environment is often offset by the difficulty of getting all the work done in the time available. If you could only chart faster—but you don't yet know how to write progress notes fulfilling all regulations. A sense of priorities is still lacking; there is always so much to do.

If seeing the light begins at 3 months, the end of the tunnel itself comes at about 6 months after orientation. By then, the nursing process is better understood, and care plans include other disciplines as well. Determining the frequency of visits on new admissions has become easier. Nurses are able to recognize multiple needs, when present. Unfortunately, the realities of cost constraints limit the areas that can be effectively pursued. Of necessity, a better sense of priorities has finally developed. The need for family involvement in the care of patients is also clear; teaching relatives is as important as teaching the patients. A full caseload can now be managed, assisted by frequent consultations with other co-workers.

Home care is forever changing. Changes in technology, rules and regulations, and treatments make up the world of home care nursing. The knowledge that there are some specific points where progress in the fundamentals of home care can be measured can encourage newcomers to persevere in the specialty, and cope with the ever-changing, ever-interesting environment. Learning also that the difficulties are part of the transition, and are not insurmountable, can give the necessary confidence for the months ahead. Experienced home care nurses can attest to it.

PITFALLS OF TRANSITION

Even as knowledge of the home care specialty is being absorbed and utilized, unsuspected difficulties sometimes arise. Whether real or perceived, these hidden dangers of autonomy, limitations, and self-doubt, can be pitfalls of the transition. They are products of the adaptation to the new milieu and the many changes that have occurred in a short period of time. Inner feelings of inadequacy may develop when nurses new to the field are first confronted by their own limitations and the many patient needs. The caregivers' willingness to help is there, but tapping into the health care system often presents problems. This chapter highlights these three areas of difficulty, and makes suggestions on how to deal with them.

Handling Autonomy Successfully

Freedom, independence, autonomy. "Freedom denotes the rightful power to act; freedom derives from positional authority, (that is, organizational expectations for the position) and from authority of expert knowledge held by professionals who occupy the position" (Batey & Lewis, 1982, p. 15). With such positive meaning, how can this autonomy be viewed as an area of difficulty? For home care nurses, independent practice is learned through significant effort over a long period of time. It should be enjoyed as a recompense for a job well done and a goal achieved. Indeed, there is great pleasure in functioning professionally, with confidence, in an environment that is not always optimum.

With autonomy, however, come more legal implications. Techniques practiced in hospitals must be adapted to the new setting. This is not always easy, but it is necessary. Considering also the number of caregivers, family members, friends or others involved in the care of one individual, nurses can also become very vulnerable to lawsuits.

There are several ways of reducing exposure to such actions, while permitting full enjoyment of the new-found autonomy.

1. Knowing thoroughly the home care standards. "They provide guidance in achieving excellence in care" (ANA, 1986, p. 1).
2. Writing precise documentation.
3. When in homes, keeping in mind the patient's safety and acting accordingly, possibly by adding other disciplines like PT and OT, or providing necessary equipment to prevent falls.
4. Following exactly the policies and procedures of the employing agency.
5. Keeping current in professional practice.

For a more in-depth look at legal considerations in home care, several nursing books offer up-to-date information. Some recent ones are listed in the bibliography. Consulting them, as well as subscribing to professional magazines, helps nurses keep abreast of changes in the field. Being informed still remains one of the best forms of protection.

A less-explored side of home care autonomy is the additional stress it can impose on an already very full daily schedule. Eight hours of time to organize at one's leisure sounds like a tremendous opportunity. Eight hours of work without anybody looking over one's shoulder can be exhilarating. But that same flexibility can become a trap and translate into fatigue unless a strong sense of priority prevails. Nurses' days are filled by visits to patients, travel, care coordination, and paperwork. There are productivity standards to be met, as determined by each agency. It is very easy to underestimate the time certain tasks take, especially where office work is concerned. A further risk, while in the field, is the very human urge to accommodate patients by doing simple errands and other tasks or even running your own errands. As will be discussed below in the section on limitations, this is another potential time trap that can put a big hole in the 8-hour schedule. These schedule leaks, taken together, can lead to increased stress due to the shortage of hours available to complete progress notes and other necessary documents.

Time management is one way around this problem. Reviewing the priorities of the day, organizing them in sequence, and completing the nursing tasks to be done each day can give a sense of accomplishment. It also gives the opportunity to really enjoy the practical side of autonomy brought about by the new job.

Limitations of Time and of the Health Care System

"So much to do, so little time." How many times have nurses used this expression in the hospital, when overwhelmed by the work ahead! That same expression can be applied to home care practice as well. It seems that there are always more tasks to complete in one day than there is time to fit them in. There are other limitations to be aware of, however, besides the time constraint. These are examined in this section on "Pitfalls" because they can be a great source of frustration for nurses new to the specialty. Being alerted to a difficulty might help decrease its intensity and save unnecessary worry.

Better time management usually helps to improve output and increase satisfaction with the day's accomplishments. However, limitations imposed by the health care system can both affect newcomers' morale and influence the plans of patient care: There are so many recognized needs, and so few resources. By the time nurses new to home care are able to fully identify the patients' needs when making home visits, they also come to realize the limitations on responding to some of them.

For example, Medicare is a medically oriented system; hence, it does not cover in-home needs, such as cleaning and shopping for the frail, the ill or the elderly. That kind of assistance, which could possibly prevent another admission to a hospital or a skilled nursing facility, is not included in the basic benefits during convalescence. Third-party payors often do not cover physical or occupational therapy, even when the safety of a patient is compromised. When confronted by a disparity of needs and resources, nurses have proven very creative in juggling those resources that are available. Using the team approach, and calling on the resourcefulness of social workers and volunteers, patients can often be provided temporary assistance for food delivery and care of pets. With the approval of patients, when even out-of-town family and friends are made aware of the patient's needs, nurses have been able to arrange more permanent solutions.

Faced daily by limitations on time and services covered, nurses must make choices. Should they go to the pharmacy to pick up a patient's new prescriptions? Should they run errands for bedridden individuals? Should they give the patient a ride to a doctor's office? Compassion is a characteristic of home care nursing. The desire to help can be very powerful at times and can result in impulsive decisions. Keeping in mind that one of the nurse's functions in home care is *to identify* the resources that will assist patients in achieving a maximum level of independence will help the nurse in making more rational decisions.

Other factors to consider are: time, safety for self, and the legality of the action one is about to take. These perspectives might assist in resolving a few dilemmas.

It has been said that "we cannot solve all problems for every patient." Sometimes, by wanting to do too much, nurses might rob patients of their independence and make them feel helpless. Optimal levels of well-being need to be met with the full participation of each individual, as mentioned in the *Homecare Bill of Rights.* It is one of the challenges of home care nursing.

Self-Doubt

Confronted by so much that is new during the transition, it is not uncommon to doubt one's own ability to absorb it all. At the same time, learning to meet the ever-elusive need for time to fit in all the tasks only compounds the difficulty. Experienced home care nurses know that things eventually fall into place, but the uncertainty can trigger an unsettling feeling in novices. "Will I ever be able to learn it all, let alone utilize the knowledge appropriately in homes?" "How can I follow the rules of asepsis in cluttered apartments?" From memorization of Medicare documentation guidelines to application of clinical skills, no subject is exempt; self-doubt is not selective.

Especially during the first few months, it is difficult to remember that there is not only one way to solve nursing problems. Learning to transfer and to adapt the skills used in hospitals to the home environment is part of mastering the new specialty. Each situation pulls from nurses' past experience and finds an application to the new milieu. Having been exposed to different degrees of acuity in hospital helps the decision-making process.

To overcome self-doubt, some of the suggestions made earlier apply:

1. Accessing resources (preceptor, supervisor, and co-workers) as often as necessary *is most important.* Paging an experienced professional for assistance whenever there is a clinical, ethical or legal question can be reassuring.
2. Discussing a nursing action in homes *each time* there is a doubt about its appropriateness will help reduce anxiety and build confidence.
3. Strict adherence to the agency's policies and procedures cannot be overemphasized.

Trying to look professional, experienced, sociable, and collected when making first home visits is hard. By keeping in mind that learning is a process, a new notion of time can be developed; it can become a friend. Feelings of self-doubt can then be recognized as only a normal part of the transition and the adaptation from the old to the new setting.

SUCCESSFUL ADAPTATION

When moving to the home care specialty from a hospital, how do you know when you have grasped the main concepts, conquered the differences, and completed the transition?

A transition is a passage, a change, and an adaptation. The ability to adapt varies for each individual. Learning to function effectively in a new environment takes time. There is no concrete point determining total control of the new specialty. However, most nurses who have made the journey feel that about 1 year after orientation is when they felt comfortable functioning independently. It was not necessarily the case that there were no more questions to ask or new situations to handle, but rather that they were able to case manage a full patient load without major difficulties.

Besides positive evaluations by supervisors, and increased participation in team conferences, there are some psychological and practical clues that indicate that the adaptation has been successful. Here are some of them:

1. Enjoying fully the daily contact with patients, in their own homes.
2. A tremendous increase in level of comfort prioritizing problems, especially when doing assessments and writing care plans.
3. Functioning autonomously; having also developed a strong support system (resources) within the agency.
4. Coming to the realization that a major role of the home care nurse is being the patients' advocate with third-party payors.
5. Appreciating, finally, the variety and flexibility of home care. By this time, hospital nursing might even have completely lost its appeal.
6. Thoroughly enjoying the freedom of scheduling one's own visits.
7. Answering questions for newcomers, and offering suggestions.
8. Accepting the fact that, in home care, the paperwork is never done.

As was discussed at the beginning of this chapter, the two major differences between hospital and home care nursing are *autonomy of decision making* and *increased responsibilities related to reimbursement.* A general feeling of having refined these skills, and of being able to apply them to everyday home situations, is really the main sign that—yes—one has successfully made the change. At this point, the distinction of being called a home care nurse has been earned. To continue to enjoy the one-to-one patient contact, the challenge to creativity by high-tech home care treatments, and to know that you are really making a difference in the lives of many—these rank high among the rewards of home care nursing.

PART II

HOME CARE NURSING PRACTICE

Chapter 4

MAKING THE HOME VISIT: FROM PREPARATION TO COMPLETION

This chapter concentrates on actual home care nursing work. In practice, achieving quality care and effective patient teaching takes the assistance of families and professionals of other disciplines. Through documentation, nurses demonstrate that their care to each individual was appropriate and effective. Accountability to consumers is a must. Ways to conquer the daily routine are suggested so that quality care can be provided and demonstrated without creating undue stress in either caregivers or patients.

The following chapter is divided into "before, during, and after," and presents the actual logistics of a home visit. It incorporates suggestions to promote understanding and to simplify the process. Good working habits, learned at the beginning, translate into timesavers. When these habits are combined with your clinical skills, no nursing challenge will be unsurmountable.

In the Albrecht Nursing Model for Home Health Care, Albrecht (1990) (see Figure 4.1), 8 variables are identified as contributing to the outcome of care at home. They are divided into 3 main components: structure, process, and outcome.

The elements of *structure* include the client, family, loved one, provider agency, professional nurse, and health team. The *process* elements include the type of care, coordination of care, and intervention. Satisfaction with care, quality of care, cost effectiveness, health status, self-care capability, and use of home care are the *outcome* elements. The successful achieve-

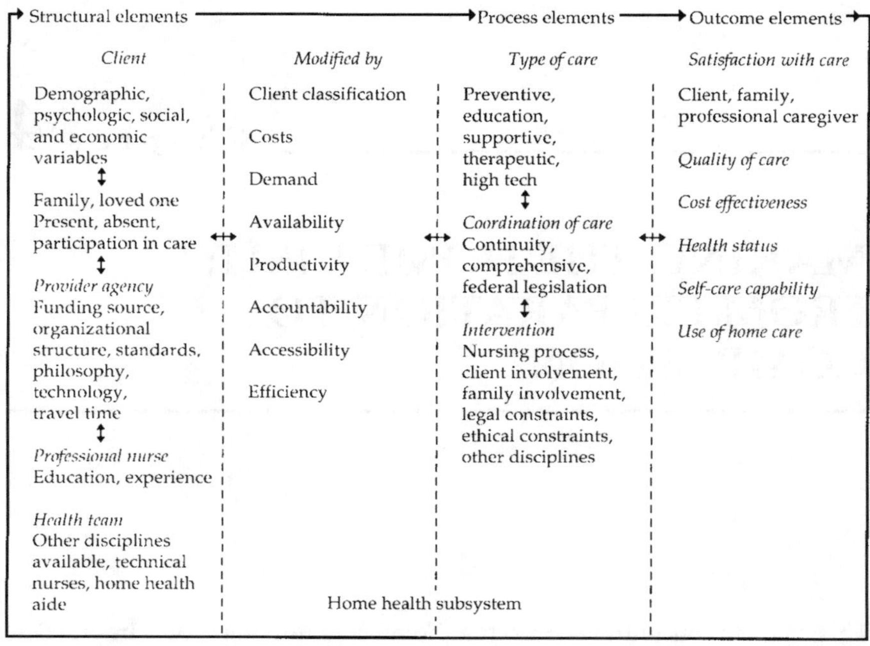

FIGURE 4.1 The Albrecht nursing model for home health care. Reprinted with permission of Blackwell Science, Inc., *The Albrecht Nursing Model for Home Health Care: Implications for Research, Practice, and Education*, by Albrecht, M. N. (1990), *Public Health Nursing*, *7*(2), p. 123.

ment of these outcomes is determined by the adequacy of the structure and process elements. The complexity of home care, and the many factors influencing the quality of the delivery, is reflected in the model. Relationships among variables and needs for in-service programs are also identified. This gives direction for research, nursing practice and education. This chapter will integrate the elements of structure, process, and outcomes.

BEFORE THE VISIT

Making your first home care visit can be an unnerving experience. Several preliminary steps can be taken to facilitate the assignment and to increase your confidence. The right information, if acquired beforehand, will permit concentration on the patient's problems, not your own worries.

This section examines the necessary preparation for a home visit. It explains sources of patient referrals and analyzes a registration sheet, the form on which all the data provided by the referral source is recorded. By focusing on a few key pieces of that input, you can have a fairly good picture of the work ahead. Information is also provided about pertinent materials to review in light of the referral data.

Referrals

Referrals to home care agencies come from many sources: physicians, podiatrists, hospital discharge planners, and social workers are some examples. Frequently, patients who feel unable to go to their MD's office call their doctors and refer themselves. The physician then telephones a home care agency and asks for an evaluation visit by a registered nurse, with instructions to report back.

Each case is reviewed individually to determine if goals can be met in the home setting. Every agency has basic admission criteria to screen patients. While those criteria may vary, one of them is mandatory everywhere: each patient must be under the care of a physician.

Information provided by the referral source is gathered on the particular agency's registration form. Data collected is basically the same: demographics, diagnoses, procedures, primary and secondary physician, if applicable, referral source, hospital or institution, with duration of stay, payor sources (reimbursement), brief clinical and psychosocial data, physician's orders for each discipline requested (registered nurse, physical, occupational, and speech therapists, social worker, Home Health Aide), and list of current medications.

Given all this information, as the admitting nurse, where do you start? What are the most important pieces? Where should you focus in preparation for the initial visit? There are several ways of analyzing the form to achieve the same results. Here is one way that I have found works well and saves time:

1. Start with the address. If your agency provides security escort service, and the address is located in a designated escort area, order the service now. You will then have more flexibility in your schedule.
2. Check the spoken language. Verify if a relative is designated or if a translator is requested. If no one in the home speaks English, find out if your agency is a subscriber to a telephone translation service, such as

AT&T Language Line®. If so, write down the 800 number and your agency's identification number. It will help in scheduling the visit and also when reaching the home.

3. What is the primary diagnosis? Was the patient hospitalized? Was there any surgery performed?

4. With the above information in mind, now read the service orders. If blood needs to be drawn, a Foley catheter is to be changed, or if any treatment has been ordered that requires supplies, order them now. Glance at the payor source, and add it to the order. By giving the storeroom clerk sufficient time, your order will be ready to go when you are.

If you gather your own supplies, as is the case in some agencies, follow the same sequence of actions. In the case of wound care, the hospital typically gives the patients enough supplies for the first few days after discharge. Verify this when calling to make an appointment. As a cost constraint measure, many hospitals are changing their policies on this subject. If for some reason there are no supplies in the home, bring 4 x 4s, tape, or whatever is required, based on the treatment ordered.

By now, you should have an overall picture of the case. Read the rest of the information, including the history if it has been provided. Following the above process yields the most information from a registration sheet in a relatively short time. It also prevents your eyes from wandering all over the page(s), gathering bits and pieces of information without focus. Every minute counts in home care, before, during or after the visits.

5. Call the patient to make an appointment. Ask: Is this the correct address? Is there an apartment number? What is the cross street? May I park in the driveway? Are you able to get to the door? If not, is there somebody available to open the door? (Most patients will let you know if there is a special way to announce yourself when at the door, i.e., "three rings.") Could you have your Medicare, Medicaid, or insurance card (whatever is appropriate) available for me to check, please if possible?

6. Arrange the forms needed in the home (see Documents) in the order they will be introduced. It will decrease the shuffling of papers, distracting to the patient and nurse alike. Fill in the patient's name and date, if time permits.

The information provided by the referral source is also very helpful at subsequent visits. It is especially important if you are not familiar with the patients and are seeing them in place of the regularly assigned case managers. The analysis does not have to be as exhaustive as described above, but a glance at the diagnosis and procedures will help you put the visit into perspective.

Review of Pertinent Material

Diagnoses vary; so does the body of knowledge and the work experience of nurses. Before a home visit, most diagnoses probably look very familiar. Others may not, due to a lack of exposure in the previous work setting. Another reason could be the recent development of new hospital procedures. Home care requires constant learning of specific new post-op care. What are the complications we should be aware of, so we can teach more effectively? In the case of a less familiar disease, what is the pathophysiology? Are there new medications? What are the side effects? Increased knowledge helps nurses and patients alike. Informed patients are more willing to participate in their care, knowing which symptoms to be aware of in case of complications, and the medication side effects to anticipate. Informed nurses feel more comfortable; consequently, when making home visits, they are better teachers. Given the time constraints of the job, especially those present in the morning when setting up a schedule for the day, how do you go about gathering the information you need?

1. *Talk with your co-workers.* Perhaps because we do not see our home care colleagues on a regular basis, we often forget what valuable resources they are. Check if they have any information on the subject you are interested in. They frequently have had a patient with a similar problem and had to do some research themselves.
2. *Consult with your supervisor.* Because supervisors have an administrative role, the tendency is to underappreciate their clinical knowledge. However, they assist their staff members in coming up with solutions to problems on a daily basis. Consequently, they have lots of exposure to a variety of situations. More often than not, they will be able to assist you or direct you to a specific resource.
3. *Check your education department.* Each agency has a collection of books and magazines. My experience is that *Nursing96, Home Healthcare Nurse,* and *RN* provide the most current information on clinical subjects. If the questions involve new medications, even the latest drug book might not have the data you are looking for. Call a hospital pharmacy or the drug information center at your closest university medical center.

Whatever the question, the better informed you are before reaching the home, the more comfortable and effective you will be when you are there. It is worth the time and effort. Eventually, you will also become a good resource for other nurses in your unit.

DURING THE VISIT

Behavior in the Home

When making home visits, "remember that you are a guest in the home. Although invited and often welcomed, you must move within the home according to the client's cues. Don't expect formal treatment. Move at a reasonable pace without rushing through questions or treatments. Note whether the client prefers to sit in a particular chair, and avoid using it yourself. If appropriate, you may wish to comment on the environment, such as 'What a lovely home,' but don't handle personal items or inquire at length about them" (Liebermann, 1990, p. 10).

Here are a few more suggestions to add to this basic code of behavior. The aim is to show respect for the patients and their property.

1. Avoid walking on lawns on the way to homes. Use walkways.
2. Never use the telephone without first asking for permission.
3. The same applies to sitting on beds. Many people consider their bed a very special area, no matter how cluttered the home.
4. If drawing blood, use a chuck or ask for an old towel to place under the arm, in case of spillage.
5. Teach in words easy to comprehend.
6. If patients are hard of hearing, talk loudly enough. It is important to evaluate whether a patient is confused, or is simply hard of hearing.
7. Do not discuss other patients' ailments or difficulties. Nobody really wants to listen to others' miseries. No matter how much less dramatic their own problems are, they are still difficult enough to handle.
8. Never call patients, especially the elderly, by their first names unless invited to do so.
9. If, on entering an Asian home, you see the occupants' shoes by the door, ask if you should follow the custom yourself.

Those rules are not complicated or difficult to follow. However, they can make a lot of difference in how people view nurses. Nursing skills and good manners must go hand in hand into the patients' homes.

Documents

At the initial home visit, several documents must be presented to the patient before the actual interview/assessment takes place. The basic documents are: *Homecare Bill of Rights*, treatment consent form, Medicare secondary-payor screening questionnaire (if patient is covered by Medicare), and Advance Directives. All these forms are requirements for home care providers. Check with your preceptor for the formats used by your agency. Read each one to become familiar with its content and its implications. They must be explained to patients. It is time-consuming. How can it be accomplished well in the least amount of time?

1. When in the home, state clearly the purpose of the visit. An easy way to accomplish this is to review with the patient some of the information provided on the registration sheet: the physician's name, reason for going to the hospital (if it is the case), length of stay, procedures done, and service orders. Doing this will help the patient feel at ease. Most importantly, it puts you in control of the time element, by preventing the patient from starting to describe an entire hospital stay with all the problems it created.

2. Present the *Homecare Bill of Rights* (refer to Part I, chapter 3, *Orientation*). The ideal way of handling this requirement is for the patient to read the entire form when presented. However, many patients have poor eyesight, are slow readers or have a short attention span; others may not be comfortable with English. For whatever reason, they may be unwilling or unable to do the reading. The best approach is to then read the document to the patient, with a few explanations as you go along.

It has been my experience that by the end of the reading, the patient will already have a sense of what visiting nurses do and don't do. It can be looked at as a general introduction to home care.

To facilitate communication, some agencies make available translations of the document in the languages most frequently used by the population they serve.

3. Verify the payor source directly from the patient's identification cards; recheck the numbers and the correct spelling of the patient's name. Ask if there is any other insurance. On admission to home care these days, many seniors are found more and more often to have turned over their Medicare benefits to a Health Maintenance Organization (HMO). Frequently, they will either have forgotten about it or will be unaware of the implications of having done so. As seen in Part I, *Reimbursement*, this has a direct effect on both the number of visits and on the supplies and equipment you can provide.

4. Explain the Treatment Consent form. Have it signed.

5. Present any other forms your agency requires.

6. Introduce *Durable Power of Attorney for Health Care: Patient Guidelines*. Since the Patient Self-Determination Act went into effect in December

1991, "At or before admission, each patient must be informed, in writing, of his right under that state's law to accept or refuse medical treatment while he is competent and to make decisions about the care he will receive if he loses competence" (Greve, 1991, p. 63).

More than likely, your agency has guidelines in the form of a pamphlet to assist in the presentation. If more information is requested, leave the pamphlet for the patient to read. Insurance permitting, request the assistance of a social worker to explain more thoroughly the advance directives, and possibly to supply the necessary forms.

Interview/Assessment

Assessment is the first step of the nursing process. This section deals with the logistics of the home interview/assessment. Every minute must be made to count, as the basic admission routine requires half again to twice the time of a regular or follow up visit. This time can be extended even farther depending on the condition of the patient, the availability of caregivers, the need for a conservator to sign the treatment consent, language barriers encountered, or treatments to be done.

There are several excellent books available on assessment. Some follow the questionnaire approach, while others present normal physical systems findings and deviations. Choose which presentation and format appeal to you.

If you feel that your assessment skills need polishing, consider a continuing education class. With home care becoming increasingly more utilized by physicians, courses on this subject are proliferating. Check with the education department of your local hospital. Many in-depth classes are offered by university hospitals and taught by nurse practitioners.

The following tips will help facilitate an interview/assessment and save a few valuable minutes.

1. Position yourself as comfortably as possible within the environment. Resist the tendency to talk when you could be observing and listening.
2. If pets are too close for comfort, handle it immediately (See Part II, Chapter 6).
3. Use the systems method for the assessment. Your agency most likely has a form for that. Follow the order presented. If your form is not detailed enough, make yourself a list of questions pertinent to each system. It prevents forgetting important data.

4. All systems should be assessed at each admission. The greater part of the questioning, however, should concentrate on the primary diagnosis. It is not unusual to discover problems not indicated on the registration sheet, for example, alteration in skin integrity or diabetes.

5. As a time-saving measure, if a patient is a diabetic, do a fingerstick blood glucose at the beginning of the assessment. If the patient is hypoglycemic and you must give milk or juice, you can fill in the time before you do another test in about 30 minutes.

6. When wound care treatments need to be initiated, ask the patient where the most convenient place to do the dressing changes will be. Place the supplies where the wound is to be dressed every day.

As you progress through the assessment and the nursing needs are identified, share them with the patient. "We can help you with this particular difficulty (name the problem here), and bring you up-to-date on the latest products available." One of the responsibilities of patients, as stated in the *Homecare Bill of Rights,* is to "participate in the plan of care." This is one example of how this can be accomplished: health professionals working with patients to meet their goals.

How much writing should actually be done in the home? As much as you can in order to save time later. However, the amount depends on how fast you write, how familiar you are with the form or the laptop used, and how much time you have before your next visit. More details on the different ways of taking notes follow in this chapter, in the section about *Documentation.*

Medications

It takes very little time in home care to realize how many medication-related problems there can be. Failure to fill prescriptions after hospital discharge, or an inability to read or understand labels, are just some of them. Patients with severe arthritis often have to wait until the nurse visits to start taking their medication because they cannot open the child-proof containers. Forgetfulness creates a problem of its own. Even the most well-intentioned persons can miss doses of important medications unless a system is put in place to remind them of prescribed frequencies. There are several methods that can be used to improve compliance. Countless articles have been written on the subject; a few are listed in the bibliography. This section concentrates on ways to handle the overall issue of medications at the initial visit, and also at subsequent visits. Because so much has to be done at the initial visit, one principle to follow when it comes to medications is to simply make the patient safe for the next 24 hours—that is, until you can return and concentrate on a more appropriate and permanent system. Here are some suggestions to facilitate and expedite the process:

1. Check all medications in the home against the hospital discharge checklist and your list obtained from the doctor, as written on the registration sheet.
2. Physically handle all bottles. Read the labels. Frequently, patients will have several bottles of the same medication, ordered at different times. Check the expiration dates.
3. In case of discrepancy, call the physician. There are, however, different degrees of urgency. For example, a discrepancy with a Colace order can wait. Leave a message. One with Coumadin or Prednisone cannot. Insist on an answer today.
4. If you sense that the patient has any difficulty with frequencies, make a new list in large characters to prevent any confusion. Ask for some small plates and set up the medication on these plates to cover the next 24 hours. Indicate with a self-stick note the time at which each should be taken.
5. If insulin is involved, and there is nobody in the home to assist, an early visit the following day will be indicated.

Here is a brief review of systems that can be used to assist patients in remembering their pills and time of administration.

Mediset®: A pill box for a full week. It is separated into compartments to hold 4 daily doses.

Clean egg cartons: Mark the hours of the day. Set out the medication every morning or for 6 days.

Calendar: Especially useful if patients are on changing doses of Coumadin or Prednisone.

Clocks or watches: Alarms can be set up, and reset for the next medication. Occupational therapists are very knowledgeable about gadgets appropriate for individual problems.

Cardboard: With a sample of each pill taped to it, this can be very useful if teaching a patient to refill own Mediset.

Once a system is in place, the actions and side effects of all medications should be explained over the next few visits. Many patients have a short attention span. Frequent and consistent teaching makes for better compliance.

It is not unusual to find several bottles of expired or duplicate medications in homes. What do you do with them?

> Pharmacists recommend that old medications be discarded. Six months after the prescription was first written is a standard time frame for Rx medications; OTC ("Over the Counter") products often have expiration dates printed on the label or container. Most drugs lose their effectiveness over time, and some, such as tetracyclines and acetaminophen, can become toxic. Any pill that cracks, chips, softens, develops an odor, or becomes discolored before its expiration date should also be discarded (Messner & Gardner, 1993, p. 52).

The authors also recommend that: "all outdated or unidentified medications should be flushed down the toilet to make sure no one else takes them" (p. 52). Have the patients discard them themselves after you have helped identify the outdated prescriptions.

Patient's Safety

Patient's safety is a major concern of nurses. The Joint Commission of Accreditation of Healthcare Organizations (JCAHO) recommends that every home care agency design a program to "manage the environment related to care provided which minimizes hazards and risks to patients and staff" (JCAHO, 1995, p. 234). Consequently, at the first visit, the safety of the premises has to be assessed. Documentation of extreme hazards needs to be included in the care plan, with appropriate and timely goals to improve the situation. Nurses are responsible for informing patients of hazards and making recommendations. Occupational therapists are very helpful in assisting to remedy certain situations relevant to safety. Often, a safety checklist is provided to nurses by their individual agencies, to assist in fulfilling this requirement. The list covers plans in case of fire, earthquake, medical emergencies, fire hazards, such as clutter blocking hallways or escape routes, electrical hazards, oxygen safety, and sharps disposal.

How do you comply with the JCAHO requirement without appearing threatening or making people feel that you are being critical of their lifestyle? Here are a few suggestions:

1. Communicate clearly the purpose of the survey and how it can benefit the patient. In certain cases, extreme clutter, for example, explain that it will be easier for nurses to carry on the prescribed treatments if the obstacles are removed.

2. Minimize the number of questions asked. Many hazards can be readily observed. For example, while washing your hands in the bathroom, look if there are grab bars in the shower, skid pads in the tub, or loose rugs on the floor.

3. Make the most of every move. If using the phone, check if emergency numbers are posted near the telephone; if there is oxygen in the home, verify that a "No Smoking" sign is posted; etc.

4. Because of the time constraints on the first home visit, some agencies have established a policy that a safety list can be checked at the second visit. Your agency will determine policy. However this is carried out, keep in mind that a safer home can reduce injuries to all, patients and caregivers alike.

Universal Precautions

In home care, all patients must be considered infectious. The chain of infection requires three elements: a source, a susceptible host, and a means of transmission. The source, or infectious agent, may include bacteria, viruses, and other microorganisms. It must then have an environment in which to grow. Many of the patients seen in home care are undergoing immunosuppressive therapies, such as irradiation or chemotherapy. Others have conditions or situations that increase their susceptibility to disease: AIDS, diabetes, chronic debilitating diseases, and postoperative procedures. These patients provide the ideal milieu for organisms to thrive.

Direct person-to-person contact, contact with blood or body fluids, with any contaminated piece of equipment, and airborne transfer are all modes of transmission of infectious agents. Good handwashing technique and the wearing of gloves, masks, eyewear, and gowns are all barriers to prevent exposure to the possibility of infection. Religious adherence to the universal precautions guidelines set forth by the Centers for Disease Control and Prevention (CDC) (see Table 4.1), and Occupational Safety and Health Administration (OSHA) will substantially decrease the risk of infection for caregivers and patients as well.

Information regarding CDC and OSHA guidelines is usually passed on during orientation and reviewed regularly with field staff. Be informed of the location of the posted policy and of the recommended supplies necessary to follow the regulations.

A basic infection control principle that is often overlooked in containing the spread of infection is the need for handwashing. Hands should be washed thoroughly with an antiseptic soap and warm water at the following times:

1. Before and after all patient contact.
2. After each contact with body fluids (for example, blood, urine, feces, any drainage from wounds, or saliva).
3. After removing gloves.

Most people are concerned with cleanliness, especially when they know that visiting nurses have contact with several patients a day. They appreciate seeing you wash your hands. However:

1. Ask permission before heading for either the bathroom or the kitchen. Leave the choice of location to the patient.
2. Always carry paper towels in the outside pocket of your nursing bag. Most agencies supply them.
3. If there are no facilities, use towelettes. Often agencies supply them to their field staff. Others offer a waterless cleanser. Whatever way you choose, as soon as running water is available, wash your hands.
4. If water rationing due to drought is a major consideration, utilize towelettes or waterless cleaner more frequently.

The nursing bag is still considered an important tool of home care nursing. However, it also has the potential for infection transmission. Each agency has a procedure called "a bag technique" to follow when making the home visit (see Table 4.2). The purpose is to maximize the use of your bag while carrying out the principles of asepsis. It consists in following specific steps in order to prevent contaminating the "clean" section of your bag. Adhering to the technique is part of infection control and its importance cannot be minimized.

The future of home care might not include a nursing bag. Individualized packaged disinfectants to be taken in a paper bag and disposed of at each home might be the way of things to come. Sphygmomanometer and stethoscope would then be the only actual tools remaining. Until then, following recommended procedures and universal precautions are today's known ways to decrease infection transmission.

Tuberculosis is on the rise, and now is even more resistant to drugs than before. Keep informed about the latest data and treatments. Protect yourself and your patients by following your agency's policies and procedures.

Medical Emergencies

One of the difficulties in the home is determining what constitutes an emergency. At what point should an ambulance be called? Should 911 or

TABLE 4.1 Universal Blood and Body Fluid Precautions as Per Centers for Disease Control and Prevention

1. All health care workers should routinely use appropriate barrier precautions to prevent skin and mucous membrane exposure when contact with blood or other body fluids of any patient is anticipated. Gloves should be worn for touching blood and body fluids, mucous membranes, or non-intact skin of all patients, for handling items or surfaces soiled with blood or body fluids, and for performing venipuncture and other vascular access procedures. Gloves should be changed after contact with each patient. Masks and protective eyewear or face shields should be worn during procedures that are likely to generate droplets of blood or other body fluids to prevent exposure of mucous membranes of the mouth, nose, and eyes. Gowns or aprons should be worn during procedures that are likely to generate splashes of blood or other body fluids.
2. Hands and other skin surfaces should be washed immediately and thoroughly if contaminated with blood or other body fluids. Hands should be washed immediately after gloves are removed.
3. All health care workers should take precautions to prevent injuries caused by needles, scalpels, and other sharp instruments or devices during procedures; when cleaning used instruments; during disposal of used needles; and when handling sharp instruments after procedures. To prevent needlestick injuries, needles should not be recapped, purposely bent or broken by hand, removed from disposable syringes, or otherwise manipulated by hand. After they are used, disposable syringes and needles, scalpel blades, and other sharp items should be placed in puncture-resistant containers for disposal; the puncture-resistant containers should be located as close as practical to the use area. Large bore reusable needles should be placed in a puncture-resistant container for transport to the reprocessing area.
4. Although saliva has not been implicated in human immunodeficiency virus (HIV) transmission, to minimize the need for emergency mouth-to-mouth resuscitation, mouthpieces, resuscitation bags, or other ventilation devices should be available for use in areas in which the need for resuscitation is predictable.
5. Health care workers who have exudative lesions or weeping dermatitis should refrain from all direct patient care and from handling patient care equipment until the condition resolves.
6. Pregnant health care workers are not known to be at greater risk of contracting HIV infection than health care workers who are not pregnant; however, if a health care worker develops HIV infection during pregnancy, the infant is at risk of infection resulting from perinatal transmission. Because of this risk, pregnant health care workers should be especially familiar with and strictly adhere to precautions to minimize the risk of HIV transmission.

Note. From Centers for Disease Control and Prevention (August 21, 1987). Recommendations for Prevention of HIV Transmission in Health-Care settings. *MMWR supplement*, volume 36, No. 2S, Universal precautions, pp. 58–68. Atlanta, GA: Author.

TABLE 4.2 Bag Technique

1. Place the bag in a clean area, preferably on a wooden table. If a clean area cannot be found, the bag should always be placed on something like a newspaper to avoid contaminating the outside of the bag. Do not place your bag on stuffed furniture or at a level where an inquisitive child or pet can gain access to the bag and contaminate it or harm themselves. Always keep your bag in sight.
2. Select something that will be used to discard contaminated equipment, such as a paper or plastic bag, or a bag made from newspaper.
3. Wash your hands using the soap and paper towels in your bag. It is always best to use your own soap and towels unless the patient has paper towels for your use. Only use a cloth towel if the client has one for your use only. If it is not appropriate to use soap and paper towels, alcohol foam and gel can be used or rubbing your hands with an alcohol sponge with great friction can be used as a last option. Leave the equipment at the sink until the end of the visit when you will need to wash your hands again.
4. Only now, after handwashing, can the nurse enter the bag and take out the equipment needed for the visit. Place the equipment on a clean paper towel.
5. Proceed with the visit and discard dirty equipment into the paper or plastic bag. If syringes are used, you should know the agency's procedure for discarding them. Check this procedure with your supervisor before making home visits. If there is an unusually large, contaminated dressing, another bag may be needed. The family should be taught how to discard all dirty equipment safely.
6. When the visit is completed, clean the used equipment with the solution(s) recommended by your agency, as based on OSHA regulations, and wash your hands before replacing equipment in the bag. Never reenter the bag unless you have washed your hands.
7. Close the bag and leave it in a clean area until you are ready to leave.

Note. From *Orientation to Home Care Nursing* (p. 46), by C. Humphrey and P. Milone-Nuzzo, 1996. Gaithersburg, MD: Aspen. Copyright 1996 by Aspen Publishers, Inc. Reprinted with permission.

the local medical emergency system be used? Even these are not always easy decisions to make, let alone knowing which ambulance company to call. For nurses who have worked in hospitals prior to home care, the many degrees of acuity experienced serve as a point of reference. The situations are familiar; it is the responses which must be relearned. What happens when 911 is called? A dispatcher determines the priority of the call and sends the fire and/or police department, if indicated. Priorities A, B, or C are then assigned, A necessitating an immediate response. It is urgent, therefore, that you identify the type of situation before you make the call. Community guidelines regarding the use of 911 are available for the asking.

In your own judgment, if a situation is critical, do not hesitate to call 911. It is better to overestimate a condition than to jeopardize a patient's life. Call the doctor immediately after handling the emergency.

If the situation is less acute, discuss the patient's condition with their personal physician. If patients need to be taken to a hospital, call an ambulance directly. Instruct them to go to the emergency room indicated by the doctor.

If you are unable to reach their regular physician, and patients need to be seen and evaluated by a doctor, have a relative or a friend drive the patient to the nearest or most familiar emergency room. In all cases, a Confirmation of Verbal Order (CVO) must be written and sent to the physician afterwards, for signature.

Which ambulance company do you call? Two questions should be asked: "How soon does the patient need to reach the hospital?" and "Which ambulance has given the best service in the past?" Initially, you may have to rely on others in the agency to answer this last question, but the answer will definitely influence your future calls. Your agency should provide you with a list of local ambulance companies. If it does not, make your own list from the yellow pages. When you need an ambulance, go down the list and ask if a vehicle is available. Choose the one with the shortest waiting period, because 30–45 minute waits are not uncommon. Often, however they arrive sooner, to the benefit of the patient.

One fine point, in these times of cost containment, is relative price. The *Homecare Bill of Rights* reminds us that patients must know in advance if they will be responsible for any costs. After inquiring about charges, inform family members.

Most private insurances require an authorization prior to calling an ambulance, unless, of course, you are dealing with a dire emergency. They will tell you if they want to use a particular ambulance company.

Whatever the urgency of a situation in a home, take time to explain to the family the reason for your course of action. Emergencies are always very traumatic; anxiety levels are high. Often, arrangements have to be made hastily so children can be taken care of. Full understanding and reassurance might not always be achievable, in view of the acuity of the moment; but there is always room for empathy.

Visit Conclusion

The assessment has been completed, the needs have been identified, and the consent has been signed. It is time to leave. The lengthy process of admission can be very tiring for the mostly elderly population we serve, even more so than regular visits. There are also different degrees of forgetfulness. Before you depart:

1. Repeat the number of the agency where you can be reached. With the patient's permission, place a sticker on the telephone.
2. Tell them when your next visit is going to be.
3. If a Home Health Aide, a social worker, or any other specialty has been added, mention it again. People usually remember the last pieces of information that have been passed on.
4. If you have moved a piece of furniture to facilitate the interview, put it back where it was. Dispose of gloves or other items you have used.
5. Keep in mind at all times that you represent nurses in general and home care in particular. The agency will be judged on your behavior in the home today.

If for some reason a patient declines further visits, do not take it personally. Many patients are very well able to take care of themselves. Inform the physician of the refusal of treatment. However, if a patient resists treatment, and in your professional judgment there is definite need, try your best to convince him or her. Point out the benefits of ongoing assessment, such as possible avoidance of rehospitalization in the near future.

AFTER THE VISIT

Working Habits

Assessment and diagnosis, the first and second phases of the nursing process, take place during the admission visit. The third phase, planning, starts in the home, but the actual writing of the care plan occurs post-visit. During the subsequent calls, implementation follows, along with ongoing evaluation.

Certain working habits, acquired at the beginning of the new career, will actually facilitate the application of the nursing process. They will also help expedite the routine, following the daily visits. The first habit that comes to mind is: should you go back to the office or go home after you have completed the day's visits? There are as many good reasons to do one as the other. Nurses who have been working in home care for a year or more are likely to complete their daily work at home most of the time. Let's look at the factors influencing choices. We know that the office is a busy, noisy place, with many interruptions. However, that is where some of the resources are: supervisors, co-workers, and clerical staff. One can get answers immediately; there are so many questions when one is beginning in home care. Another reason to return to the office is ready access to forms of all kinds. On an ordinary day, a variety of forms is needed, in addition to regular progress notes, to fulfill Medicare and other insurance requirements.

After particularly stressful fieldwork, the office is the place to go if one needs to discuss the events of the day. More experienced nurses, remembering their own first few months in home care, are always very supportive.

Home, however, is a quieter place to do charting. Concentration is facilitated. Phone calls to physicians, supply companies, and laboratories can be made as well from the home as the office. Being available to make appointments with plumbers, electricians or delivery persons is one of the great advantages of working from home.

Based on the author's experience, the initial recommendation for nurses new to home care is to return to the office after seeing patients. The quick access to resources is crucial, especially for the first 5 to 6 months. Later, when working from home, remember that charts of patients who must be visited during the weekend need to be returned to the office on Friday. Wherever nurses end up at the end of the day, it is their choice. It shows again how flexible home care can be.

Another working habit to develop, a great timesaver after home visits, is automatic followup tasks. The best way to accomplish this is to repeat the same sequence of actions over and over again, day in and day out. As an example, on returning to the office after seeing patients:

1. *Head directly for the secretary's desk.* Indicate which patients were seen, by whatever method the agency chooses.
2. *Go to your desk.* Check messages, telephone, voice mail or faxes.
3. *Complete your checklist for the day.*

Such a sequence of tasks, as banal as it sounds, will most easily accomplish what needs to be done. The more mechanical these tasks become, the faster and more surely you will complete them in the future. Getting these things out of the way first will also reduce panicky feelings caused by the sight of the new memos, communication notes, and charts dropped on your desk in your absence.

It has been said at time management lectures: "Handle every piece of paper only once." This advice surely applies to home care work. When writing progress notes or doing admissions, pick up each form and try to complete it as thoroughly as possible. Concentrate. It is really worth the effort. As time goes on, the forms themselves will become more familiar and you will have more time to focus on your answers. If there are unanswered questions along the way, and nobody is available for consultation, place a self-stick note at the location and complete as much of the page as possible. Later, when you ask for help with the difficulties, the form will then be complete.

Be on guard against the tendency to procrastinate. Postponing the writing of forms such as Confirmations of Doctors' Verbal Orders (CVOs) that were called in by telephone that day is a step backwards. The recollection of the clinical findings takes twice as long in the following days. The facts are not fresh, and accuracy is very important. CVOs are legal documents. A golden rule to follow is: if it takes only 5 minutes, do it now.

Telephone Priorities

So much to do! Where should I start? Whether finishing up at the office or at home, after that day's visits are completed, some priorities remain the same. Telephone calls are first on the list. The more calls made from the patients' homes, the better, as far as timesaving goes. One should be cautious in calling from the patient's home, however; at times, it may be inappropriate to discuss the condition in front of the patient. Some calls have to wait because of time constraints between visits, or the need to be near a telephone to receive an answer within a given time.

1. If blood was drawn early in the day, a call to the laboratory to get the results should be made first.
2. Calls to physicians come next. Leave messages, if necessary, including your beeper number. Should there be blood values to report that might result in a change of medication, do it quickly. The patient might still need to be contacted that day, to be made aware of the change. Calling doctors early gives them more time to return the calls before the end of the day.
3. If authorizations from insurance companies are needed for further home visits or supplies, these calls come next.
4. Finally, call supply companies if equipment is needed and patients have been informed of costs, as pointed out in the *Homecare Bill of Rights* (see Part I, Table 2.2).

I would like to stress the importance of leaving messages. When you are unable to reach someone, calling back without leaving a message may seem to be the thing to do. After all, it takes time to leave one's name, plus all the information to be passed on, let alone spelling every word. However, it takes more time to call later. It also interrupts the writing of progress notes and the flow of ideas. Even worse is the possibility of forgetting to call back. Leave messages. Be forceful. Clear and concise messages are very effective. Most importantly, briefly jot down who was called (by name), when, for what reason, and who took the message. The mind is now free to concentrate on the paperwork.

It is also a good habit to learn to send short notes to persons who were particularly helpful in an emergency. Everyone likes to be appreciated. It is good public relations for home care nurses and for their agency, not to mention an improvement to everyone's working environment.

Documentation

In the business of home care, documentation is the product. As all nurses learn from day one, if it isn't charted, it isn't done. It is the means of communication between the home care nurse in the field and the supervisor. It is what provides the basis for continuity of care. It provides legal protection in case of question or dispute. Finally, it is the source of reimbursement.

Not surprisingly, then, documentation takes a major part of your workday. The good news is that the process does quickly become easier as the forms and terminology become more familiar. Your chart will reflect all interactions in the home, with patients and family, teaching, and training, as well as direct care. As always, there are guidelines:

1. The record must be accurate in all respects.
2. The actual content of the record should contain measurable and objective information rather than subjective statements.
3. Initial and ongoing assessments and nursing interventions must be documented in the record.
4. In the home care situation it is important not only to document direct observations, but to indicate what was taught to family members and the client in order to ensure proper monitoring of his condition (Humphrey & Milone-Nuzzo, 1996, pp. 81–82).

To facilitate the documentation process, this section concentrates on the actual logistics of writing progress notes, rather than principles of effective documentation. There are several ways charting can be done, based on your home care experience and preference.

1. Charting on the actual progress notes, in the patients homes, as the data is being gathered. However, especially at first, it is difficult to concentrate on the patient, learn the skills of interviewing, do treatments, and

chart, all in a totally new environment. Further, the patient is likely to feel ignored if too much time is spent writing. This method can be saved for later, when you feel more comfortable in the home. If your agency provides laptop computers, the same procedure can be followed.

2. Using self-stick notes in the home is the recommended practice at the beginning. The actual charting can be done later, perhaps in the car, immediately after the visit.

Dictation is also utilized by some agencies; the data is transcribed later at the office, by a special team, and added to the chart.

It takes discipline to follow through immediately with documentation, but it is more than worth the effort. One good reason to drive away before charting would be if the visit was in an unsafe area of town. Even then, on the way to the next appointment, it is recommended that you drive to a safer neighborhood, park, and chart while the ideas are fresh. Another possible reason for postponing charting would be if you were accompanied by a security guard during the visit. The guard's time is also valuable; there is usually another commitment waiting. Again, after being dropped off at your car, you can chart before driving away. If, however, the visit was for the admission of a new patient, recording the greater amount of data may have to be saved for later, when sufficient time is available.

Learning to process an admission takes concentration. It also takes the preceptor's assistance. If visits have been scheduled too close to each other, and time commitments would otherwise not be met, complete the visits, take notes, and save the charting for later.

Whichever method of charting is selected, there is a way to save some minutes, even when inspiration is lacking. In order to get the momentum going, start writing, even if it is only your name at the end of the page, the date, or the time of the visit. Do not interrupt the flow. Concentration will prevent the mind from wandering and will re-stimulate the ideas. It does work.

A list of acceptable medical abbreviations is usually provided to new home care nurses during orientation. Taking time to learn them will eventually shorten charting.

How are priorities determined when noting nursing problems on a new treatment plan? Every agency has its own form to gather information on admission. It could be a multiple-choice and checkmarks form or a review of systems with narrative descriptions. Whatever method is used, it should incorporate the eligibility criteria for Medicare: care under the direction of a physician, intermittent, skilled, reasonable and necessary, and homebound status to justify reimbursement, as seen in Chapter 2, under *Reimbursement*. Once these criteria are established, listing the nursing problems is easier:

1. Look at the primary diagnosis on the registration sheet. Based on the assessment, sometimes the secondary diagnosis becomes primary. Feel free to reverse the order, if appropriate. The first problem listed should be related to the primary diagnosis. If more than one diagnosis is listed, review your assessment to see if you found current problems related to them.
2. List other alterations in systems status.
3. Are there knowledge deficits? They come next.
4. Psychosocial problems and safety issues are also mentioned in the care plan, often listed at the end.

This is one way of listing problems. As you become more acquainted with the forms and have more experience in the field, this sequence can be changed as needed.

Considering how difficult it is to define and list problems, this method simplifies the process, at the beginning. Several books are on the market to assist home care nurses with documentation. I have also found books labeled "patient teaching guides" very helpful in identifying problems.

Other Specialties

One of the goals of home care is to make the patient as independent as possible. To accomplish this, nurses need help. Every agency has a number of specialists available, including physical, occupational, and speech therapists. When should you call on these, or other specialties, if the referring physician has not already made a request? Think "safety in the home." Some general guidelines follow regarding each specialty:

Physical Therapy

These specialists place an emphasis on mobility, strength, balance, and safety. Pain control and cardiac rehabilitation.

Occupational Therapy

Here the emphasis is on Activities of Daily Living (ADLs), energy conservation, and adaptive aids.

Speech-Language Pathology (Speech Therapy)

These specialists place an emphasis on dysphagia of any kind and recent onset of change in voice.

Social Work

Social workers bring a special kind of assistance to new home care nurses. Sometimes, it is very difficult to separate the social or emotional problems from the true health problems. "Depending on their severity, social problems can adversely affect a patient's response to a specifically prescribed medical regimen, rendering it less effective than desired, or even totally ineffective" (*Medicare Health Insurance Manual–11,* 206.1). Consequently, it is important to seek the guidance of Medical Social Workers (MSWs) to help make sense of these particularly complicated home situations. Early utilization of this resource can both save nursing time and speed patient recovery. The MSW's focus on specific community agencies for patient referral can be particularly helpful. MSWs offer a wealth of information to the newcomer and the home care veteran alike.

Nurse Specialists

Determining the severity of a particular health problem can be difficult. At what point should a consultation with a nursing specialist be called for? Diabetic, enterostomy, respiratory, psychiatric, and nutritional experts are available in many agencies. In case of doubt, call on them, even if the problems encountered are minor. Early intervention can save them, and the patients, many extra hours of treatment. Prevention is a large part of home care. Medicare and other insurers are also appreciative of the savings brought about by attentive nurses. This builds long-term rapport and support for future requests.

Home Health Aides

They are an important part of the home care team. Medicare has specific guidelines as to their service. Do not hesitate to call on them when patients need assistance with personal care. Aide time in each home is limited, but it is amazing how much work can be done within this time frame. These aides are trained specifically to handle the sick in home environments.

For each referral made to other disciplines:

1. A doctor's order is needed.
2. The Medicare guidelines must be followed, or
3. An authorization from private insurances must be obtained prior to the evaluation visit.

Physicians

"The patient must be under the care of a physician who is qualified to sign the physician certification and plan of care" (*Medicare Health Insurance Manual*–11, 204.3). Home care nurses could not function without them. When, then, is it appropriate to call physicians regarding their patients? Should they be called regularly for an update?

Clearly, communication between nurses and physicians is necessary. Most doctors are appreciative of the assistance provided in the homes by the nurses who monitor their postoperative patients and teach them how to take care of themselves. Preventive care at home might also save their patients further hospitalization. Why, then, are physicians so difficult to reach when needed?

Doctors and home care nurses are always on the move. Messages are passed on, then both parties move away. Beepers help, but telephones are not always handy. Not all physicians carry beepers. But, talk to each other, nurses and physicians must! Here are some general guidelines as to when you should contact doctors, in cases other than emergencies:

1. Always after admitting a patient, to notify of the start of care and clarify any order necessary. If there is no need for the physician to call back, after a message is given to the secretary, say so: "This is for information only; no need to call back unless the doctor has a question."
2. When the condition of the patient changes and necessitates a review of the orders.
3. After 62 days from admission, when the recertification is due, to review the treatment plan and make necessary changes.

One way to save time when calling physicians is to have a list of questions ready in front of you, with the name of the patients in question. It prevents shuffling papers to associate the patient and the problem. Self-stick notes placed on the chart cover work wonders. Being prepared makes you sound more professional and triggers a better response from physicians. It helps, especially if one is lucky enough, one day, to have a physician answer his/her own phone. It does happen. Leave messages at the doctors' offices early in the day, if possible. It gives you more time to call again, later in the afternoon, if there is no response.

Communication between physicians and home care nurses would greatly improve if, some day, MDs could bill for the time spent on the phone discussing their patients condition and problems. Patients would benefit, treatments would be implemented sooner, and problems would be resolved faster. Now they cannot. Therefore, the foregoing suggestions, designed to make it quicker and easier for the physician, should be very useful to nurses new to home care.

Nonbillable Visits

There are times when home care nurses make visits to patients' homes, after prior arrangement, and no one answers the door. These visits are called nonbillables. Home care agencies bill Medicare, Medicaid, and private insurers on a per-visit basis. In the case of nonbillables, because there has been no interaction between nurses and patients, the visits cannot be reimbursed.

Your agency, naturally, would like to avoid this. An even greater area of concern with nonbillables, however, is the safety of the patients. If an elderly patient agrees to see a nurse at a stated time and does not answer the door, there may be something wrong. Could it be that this patient has fallen and cannot reach the phone? Maybe the condition of the patient has worsened and necessitated a visit to an emergency room. Whatever the reason, it must be investigated. Every patient has to be accounted for.

In the event of nonbillables, you must try to find out as much as possible from neighbors or relatives. A call to physicians might be necessary. A relative or a landlord might need to be called to unlock a door. If a fall is suspected, calling the police department to break in could be the thing to do, especially if a patient has always been faithful in keeping their appointments.

Sometimes, nonbillable visits are unavoidable. Some patients do not have phones. Nurses must take a chance, go to the home, and hope to find the patient there. If there is no one home, leave a note in the mailbox or under the door. Identify yourself, indicate the time you will return, and leave the phone number of the agency, in case the patient wants to reach you. The same procedure can be followed when visiting patients in hotels where there is no phone in the rooms. Leave a message at the front desk, giving the same information as above. Ideally, your agency will have a form designed for this purpose.

Some nonbillable visits can be avoided by calling the patient's emergency contact listed on the registration sheet. Patients could be staying with relatives temporarily and have failed to mention it when they were discharged from the hospital. It could also be that patients originally scheduled for discharge that day are still hospitalized. Calling the hospital, in the case of a new admission, is a good move.

The more information gathered before setting out on the road, the more time saved. Every call made, and other attempts to reach a patient, should be documented in the chart. Nonbillables are time-consuming. Lots of effort, telephone calls, and travel time are involved.

WEEKEND WORK

The weekend and holiday experience is somewhat different from that during the week. Most patients are unfamiliar to you because they are randomly assigned from the entire agency. The number of patient visits in a day is usually higher, and concentrated more on tasks instead of caseload management. Weekend work can be rewarding and fulfilling if time is managed well throughout the day. Keep in mind that, given a choice, many weekend patients would prefer their leisure as much as you, if it were not for the required and necessary daily treatments.

Who selects the patients to be seen during the weekend? Case managers do. The needs are identified: daily wound care, monitoring of blood glucose, IV administration of antibiotics, etc. Then a special request is passed on to the weekend supervisor. Other patients call in with problems such as leaking Foley catheters or difficulty with tube feedings. All the requests are then divided and assigned to the nurses scheduled. Every agency has rotation guidelines regarding frequency of weekend work. Here are a few suggestions to assist in making the most of weekend and holiday work:

1. *Hit the road as early as possible,* as soon as assignments are completed and appointments are confirmed with patients.
2. *Keep a tight schedule.*
3. *Keep moving.*
4. *Chart after each visit.* The only chart that can wait till later in the day is writing of a new patient's care plan.
5. *Concentrate on tasks assigned.* Do not get involved with other problems unless there is an emergency or an important change in patient condition. Respect the primary relationship of the other caseworker involved.

Time passes quickly when working weekends and holidays. There is also less traffic, which makes it easier to reach patients' homes. You might even discover new parts of town. Wherever your assignment takes you, enjoy the day. Most importantly, realize that patients are insecure when professional offices are closed and the regular caseworker is not there, and anxieties are high. The tasks you perform today will be particularly appreciated.

Chapter 5

IMPORTANT ISSUES IN CASELOAD MANAGEMENT

"Caseload management is actually a managing technique so nurses can use time to deliver quality nursing care in the most effective manner at the lowest cost" (Anglin, 1992, p. 26). Each nurse's caseload is built up gradually over a period of time. As orientation progresses, new patients are added until the agency's productivity standard is reached, usually at a caseload of between 25 and 30.

Learning to meet the needs of each individual patient, while keeping a handle on the entire group, is a challenge. Spending the least amount of energy for the most results is a skill. As such, it can be learned.

Primary care, managed care, whatever method of care delivery is in place at your agency—some core responsibilities remain the same. This chapter provides information about those responsibilities as they relate to caseload management. It also includes a few suggestions on how to facilitate the execution of these duties.

RESPONSIBILITIES

Care Planning

As noted in previous chapters, every patient admitted to home care has an individual nursing care plan developed at the first visit. Specific needs, including the psychosocial ones, form the basis of the plan. A primary nurse, or case manager, is then assigned. How do you coordinate the group of patients so that each individual need is met as your caseload builds?

1. Start with each patient. Contract with each one at your first visit: "This is what we can do for you, or how we can help you, with your participation." Prioritize needs. A word of caution: resist the temptation to totally reorganize your patients' lives, or change their lifestyles. Keep in mind that the goal is simply to assist in achieving maximum independence.
2. Be clear, and also realistic, about short-term and long-term goals. Be very explicit when discussing them with each patient.
3. When assigned a patient who has been on the service for a while, review the original goals, assess what has been accomplished so far, and see what remains to be done. Then follow the procedure as above. You can't use the shortest route if you don't know where you are going. As home care gets closer to using diagnostic-related groups (DRGs) in formulating care plans, the time frame necessary to reach goals will become even more critical.
4. Organize, in whatever way works for you. The purpose is efficiency, effectiveness, and timesaving; it will also help in meeting deadlines. Here are a few suggestions:

- Keep a master list of all your patients, with due dates of recertification of treatment plans (documents due every 62 days for each patient and sent to physicians for confirmation and signature), and aides supervision (due every 2 weeks);
- Review your list at the beginning of each week, and make a note of what is due that week;
- On the front of each chart, make a list of due dates as above, including blood draws and doctor's appointments;
- Each time you write progress notes, refresh your memory by adding at the end of the note an indication of when specific tasks are due.

Caseload management goes beyond task accomplishment and paperwork. It demands autonomy of decision making and independent practice. Every day, it reminds you that good organization and follow-through are necessary to bring care plans to life. The greatest reward for your careful planning and teaching is to see your patients respond, and their conditions improve.

Case sharing might be indicated at times:

1. In the case of a patient with multiple problems, when you have been the primary nurse for quite a while, it is easy to lose perspective. By sharing the case with another nurse, you bring in a second opinion and assis-

tance in reassessing the direction of the care. Sharing can be done either by alternating visits, or dividing the tasks. The two of you can decide, based on the difficulties involved.

2. Daily visits to an individual over a long period of time, as in wound care, can be very tiring both mentally and physically. Dividing visits with another nurse might also help you keep perspective and avoid missing any subtle but important changes in a patient's condition.

If you feel that you have exhausted all your options with a particular patient that you have been following for a long time, make a request to pass on the case to another nurse. Again, bringing in someone with a new perspective might help both you and your patient.

Care Coordination

The many people and functions involved in each patient's care must all be coordinated. This is the second major responsibility of the caseload manager. The manager must knit together all of the activities involved in the different aspects of that care; for example, following up to see if the social worker has qualified the patient for food stamps. Did the supply company exchange the broken bed siderail? Was the order for the alternating pressure mattress faxed by the MD's office to the supply company? Was the wound consult done? Based on the plan of care established on admission, various orders may be given and actions taken that will demand follow-up. For example, Protime, and Lithium level need to be drawn at regular intervals; are they already ordered, or do you need to call the doctor? Also, with every additional discipline involved in the care, the need for coordination increases. Keeping in mind the specific goals for each patient helps keep you on track. It might also prevent you from overdoing and falling into the trap of trying to reorganize your patient's life.

Conferences, supervision, and discharges are all pertinent to care coordination. A brief look at each of these activities follows.

Conferences

Effective communication is a must for proper caseload management. Due to the number of health professionals involved at various times in the care of a single patient, regularly scheduled interdisciplinary conferences must take place. Because of the nature of home care, the logistics of getting everyone together to discuss those patients is a difficult task. Home care agencies' regulatory bodies understand the difficulty and have established requirements to ensure communication between disciplines. Once a month, and more often if problems arise, each care manager must touch base with the specialists also involved in their cases to discuss the plans of care, and possible changes to improve outcomes. Documentation of each conference, with the names of the participants, subject matters discussed, and changes, if any, must all be recorded.

Supervision

If your agency utilizes licensed practical nurses, also called licensed vocational nurses in some states, they must be supervised by registered nurses. There are no Medicare guidelines as to frequency. The main responsibilities of the RN in terms of supervision are making sure that the agency's policies are followed, and the plan of care for each patient adhered to.

As part of medical treatment plans, aides are frequently assigned to do personal care for specific patients. For certification and accreditation standards, home care regulatory agencies require an evaluation visit by a health professional at the patient's home every 2 weeks (for example, by a registered nurse, physical therapist, or a speech therapist, depending which discipline is managing the care). The purposes of the visits are to evaluate the quality of care provided by the aide, to assess if the plan of care is being followed, and to determine patient satisfaction with the service. Monthly, an onsite supervisory visit must be made with the aide present. The intervention, including any instruction given to the aide, needs to be documented in the progress notes.

To comply with the regulations and facilitate supervision, various evaluation tools have been developed by individual home care agencies. They measure patient outcome and evaluate the performance of tasks by the aide. Check if a form is available for that purpose at your agency.

Home care aides in general really enjoy the close contact with patients, and the opportunity to help. It is a good practice to recognize a particularly dedicated and helpful worker. By writing a simple note of thanks for a job well done, you can both acknowledge your appreciation and ensure that quality of care for the future. It is a simple step, but it goes a long way towards improving relationships in the working environment.

Discharges

As in hospitals, plans for discharges in home care are made on admission. Even with guidelines provided by Medicare, it is not always easy to determine which direction to take when planning discharges. Is the patient able to function independently? Should they remain on your service for long-term management? Critical pathways, which are standardized care plans, list a predetermined number of visits for each diagnosis. Because of their constraints, they might dictate the number of visits before a patient can be discharged, but the final decision as to appropriateness and course of action still remains the physician's, based on your input.

All goals having been met, patients can be discharged from home care services. Medically stable patients without formal support systems can be transferred to other management teams. Your best source of information regarding the diversity of agencies managing elder care is social workers. They can make recommendations based on the patient's age, mental status, needs, support system, or even respite needs of caregivers.

Patients with complex medical problems may remain under your care, indefinitely, covered under what Medicare calls "management and evaluation." If choosing that alternative, "Your assessment identification should take into consideration the following:

- Cultural and/or language barriers to traditional care
- Multiple caregivers in the home
- Caregiver's level of participation
- No caregivers in the home
- Dysfunctional caregivers
- Caregiver limitations
- Home setting that is unsafe
- Patient's reliance on multiple/complex equipment
- Need for complex services
- Involvement of multiple community resources
- History of multiple re-hospitalizations
- Multiple medical problems

The presence of some of the above are indications that management and evaluation intervention may be required" (Blue Cross of California, 1993, pp. 11–12).

When planning discharges, always remember to involve patients and family in the process. Whatever course of action you choose, your documentation must support it. The physician must also approve it. Because of frequent changes in Medicare rules and regulations, especially in view of reimbursement, check with your supervisor regarding the current policies.

Sometimes it is difficult to "let go" of certain patients. Over time, you have developed a great relationship. The atmosphere was just right for teaching or to carry out treatments; the visits were always enjoyable. How do you handle it? Remind yourself that one of the main goals of home care is to make patients as independent as possible. Obviously, you have done a good job; the goals have been met. Congratulate yourself. If your patients are being transferred to hospice, occasional visits might facilitate the transition. Whatever happens, remember the good days and go on. Other patients are waiting for your expertise.

CONFIDENTIALITY

Confidentiality, a patient's right to privacy, is an established principle of the Nursing Code of Professional Ethics (American Nurses Association, 1985). That right to privacy extends confidential status to both clinical and personal information about the patients and their families. Confidentiality can be introduced to the patients when explaining the *Homecare Bill of Rights:*

> Clients have the right: to confidentiality of the medical record as well as information about their health, social, and financial circumstances and about what takes place in the home; and to expect the home care provider to release information only as required by law or authorized by the client and to be informed of procedures for disclosure (National Association for Home Care, 1993, p. 1).

Under Medicare regulations, no information can be released without the patient's written consent. That permission is requested on the admission visit.

The subjects of confidentiality and home care legal considerations are usually covered at length during orientation. Be informed of your agency's policy regarding disclosure of medical information, and also documentation of HIV-positive patients.

As an element of caseload management, there are precautions that can be taken to maintain your patients' confidentiality:

1. At the office, keep charts not in use in your desk drawer or otherwise unexposed. Retrieve fax-transmitted documents as soon as possible after receipt.
2. Refrain from discussing patients in elevators, coffee rooms, and other public places.
3. In your car, do not leave charts exposed with names and addresses showing. This precaution is even more critical if patients' house keys are attached to the charts.
4. When working at home, do not permit access to the charts to your

family or friends. The same applies to information in computer files. Do not give out your computer password to anybody.

5. During visits, guard against the accidental exposure of other patients' confidential data.

6. Avoid unguarded comments to friends, family, or neighbors that might in any way infringe on this important right to privacy.

Because of the variety of situations home care nurses experience, it is sometimes tempting to relate specific incidents to people outside the field. Confidentiality applies to those stories also, no matter how tempting disclosure may be. Keep in mind that the world is small and listeners of yours might know the people involved. That thought, and recognition of the embarrassment disclosure would bring, should help maintain your discretion in preserving that most precious right that is confidentiality.

QUALITY ASSURANCE

Standards of practice are guidelines to ensure that quality care is being provided to consumers. They identify appropriate nursing conduct in specific situations. Nurses are accountable, to their patients and to their employing agency, for upholding these standards, and for providing high-quality nursing care.

Home care agencies, like hospitals, have programs in place to measure the quality of care. Accreditation by regulating bodies, Joint Commission on Accreditation of Healthcare Organizations (JCAHO), Community Health Accreditation Program (CHAP), and National Home Caring Council, is the seal of approval and the reward for compliance with those strict regulations. What does quality assurance mean to you as a caseload manager?

As noted in Chapter 1, standards of care are integrated throughout the policies and procedures of your agency. For example: explaining rights and responsibilities to patients on admission, writing measurable goals, and following bag technique are just some of the actions to be performed to meet standards. Several of the requirements for accreditation have time frames. In California, physicians' orders must be signed within 20 working days, as must the Confirmation of Verbal Orders, which are the orders written after the original treatment plan has been signed. Home Health Aide supervision must be documented every 2 weeks. Every state or county will have its own requirements regarding services. Besides providing the best care you are capable of, meeting these deadlines for documenting that care will do a lot towards establishing compliance with those standards.

Are your patients affected by delays in completing the paperwork on time? A treatment plan not written within 24 hours after the requested admission date might mean that no goals, short or long, have been established and documented for those particular patients. As a consequence, there might be delay in starting treatments. Infection might develop in wounds, possibly slowing down healing processes or prolonging convalescence. A delay of blood glucose or prothrombin time monitoring might also cause potentially severe problems. Those are just a few examples of factors that can affect the quality of the care you provide to your patients.

Quality assurance programs evaluate the work already done, find the most often missed areas, and concentrate on improving them through inservices to the staff. Another movement, called Continuous Quality Improvement (CQI), concentrates on prevention rather than cure. It rewards workers for their contribution to quality and efficiency. Until such time as you have become familiar with the rules, regulations, policies, and procedures in home care, some deficiencies are expected. Your best approach is this: as each new rule is encountered, memorize it and try to put it into practice immediately. "Do it right the first time" (Foreman, 1993, p. 32). Following this motto will prevent a lot of problems and wasted time fixing what should have been done correctly in the first place. Time being always at a premium in home care, this will allow you to spend that time effectively managing your caseload and providing the high-quality care for which you are valued.

RESOURCES

Understanding your resources—the sources of information, support, and assistance—and how to access those resources is fundamental for effective work. No one need stand alone when making critical decisions. As opposed to the hospital setting, where consultants are readily at hand, in home care nursing you have to look further for assistance. Lots of time and difficulty can be saved by knowing who and where to ask.

This section describes specific resources, offering suggestions based on my own experience. Clinical nurse specialists, oncology nurses, or any other professionals with whom you have worked and had a good relationship can also be good resources. The main criterion in determining a useful source is quick access: Who can I call *now* for prompt assistance with my immediate problem? The list can be as long as you want.

Co-workers

Your most accessible and understanding resources are your co-workers—Accessible, because they all carry beepers; Understanding because, at one time or another, they will have dealt with a similar situation in someone's home. They can thus relate to the difficulty you are currently experiencing.

This applies to supervisors as well. They have experienced field work and can advise you on both the legality and practicality of various courses of action. Many agencies have specialty teams such as diabetic, respiratory, wound care, or psychiatry. If you are not personally acquainted with the team members, ask the office secretaries to page one for you, and have that nurse return the call in the home where you are. These resources cover nursing and procedural questions, as opposed to medical emergencies, in which you need to contact physicians immediately. Back at the office, reviewing the immediate situation with co-workers, brings new ideas and perspectives. How else could the problem have been approached to achieve the desired results? To become proficient at home care you must keep an open mind and never hesitate to ask questions. This process is also a good way to develop trusting and long-lasting relationships with other employees in all disciplines.

Social Workers

As pointed out in Chapter 4 under *Other Specialties*, social workers bring a special kind of assistance to new home care nurses. In complicated home situations, when you feel that the psychosocial problems of your patients will interfere with their recovery, call on social workers. They are your primary source of information on issues from conservatorship to Social Security Disability regulations. They can arrange transportation to medical care, chemotherapy or radiation treatments, provide talking books for the visually challenged, and arrange assistance with medical emergency systems, meal deliveries, or even finances, to name just a few of their capabilities. In an emergency, they can even come up with food boxes for patients just discharged from the hospital who have no one to go grocery shopping for them.

Counselling and referral to support or activity groups is not beyond their job description. Their knowledge of community resources is invaluable. Check with your agency for a list of criteria for referring a patient or family for social work intervention. For each referral made, a doctor's order is needed, and the need for the discipline must be well-documented. If the patient has a private insurance, an authorization must be obtained prior to the visit.

Nurse Epidemiologists

When faced with questions or situations relating to tuberculosis, infection control, or universal precautions in homes, think "nurse epidemiologists." They can be found in hospitals. However, be it in hospitals or in patients' homes, they look for opportunities to educate. My experience is that they are quick to respond when being paged and that they refer you to reliable sources if they don't have the answer themselves.

Policy and procedure manuals are also accessible reference sources at the agency's office. Respiratory isolation in the home setting, waste disposal, and specimen handling are discussed and guidance is provided. Those books are usually found in the education department and in each supervisor's office.

Hospital Pharmacists

Hospital pharmacists are more than willing to assist with questions regarding medication interactions, clinical consequences, or any other concerns. In view of the growing utilization of generic drugs, and the difficulty of finding drug books with current information, the need to double-check unfamiliar medications is even more pressing. One drawback is that pharmacists have their own priorities, and their time is very valuable. A few university pharmacies have taken on the responsibility to fill the need and relieve other pharmacists. They have set up 24-hour information centers for health professionals and the public at large. Check with your closest university medical center to see if this service is provided.

Agency Medical Director

Most home care agencies have a medical director. Their main function is to advise the staff as to courses of action in difficult home medical situations. They also serve as the intermediary between staff and other physicians when problems arise. Before calling the director, it is a good practice to discuss the case in question with the supervisor and all other disciplines involved. Often, an answer will come during the discussion, and the call to the medical director can be avoided.

In general, the medical directors also have their own practices. The best way to access them is to leave a message at their office stating the nature of the problem.

COMMUNICATIONS

Good communication is crucial, especially in home care. You need to contact patients, physicians, co-workers, supervisors, and insurance companies throughout the day; they must be able to reach you as well. Medicare regulations require that conferences with other team members must take place at regular intervals. You are constantly on the move during working hours; so are the other team members. Yet everyone must be accessible. What are the best ways of communicating when working in the field?

Beepers

In most agencies, all personnel working in the field carry a beeper. They can sometimes become a lifeline. When difficult or unexpected situations arise in homes, and the immediate assistance of the supervisor or co-workers is needed, it is the beeper that ensures that connection. Minutes later, advice reaches the field wherever you may be, relieving anxiety for both the nurse and patient. The quick answer can be very reassuring; it helps to know that your course of action was appropriate. If used improperly, however, beepers can sometimes get in the way of your work. Every home care nurse remembers more than once having to get off the freeway to answer a call that was less than urgent. You must be accessible, but not so accessible that the temptation of turning the instrument off is irresistible. In case of doubt about a course of action, *do* use your beeper. As your orientation to home care progresses, and your confidence grows, other ways of communicating will also be appealing.

Cellular Phones

For certainty of communication, cellular phones provide even greater immediacy. Unfortunately, not all agencies offer the luxury of cellular phones for each member of their field staff. However, nurses working in rural areas or covering a sparse and large territory are sometimes given one as a timesaving device. In these cases, reimbursement for work-related calls is usually provided by the agency.

The appeal of this handy tool is such that even without the instrument or reimbursement being provided by their agencies, some nurses and therapists are buying their own. According to them, the time saved in contacting and receiving the calls back from physicians, while on the road, has been invaluable. Also, having another way to reach patients who do not respond to their front doorbell helps tremendously to reduce the stress level of these health professionals. While these calls can be tax-deductible, it is still the increased cost of air time, rather than of the instrument itself that has limited acceptance to date.

Voice Mail

A final alternative to beepers, if an answer can wait, is voice mail. The larger the home care agency, the more likely you are to find it in place. It is a communication system that permits leaving verbal messages for anyone at the agency. Special numbers also allow the system direct communication with beepers, if needed. The advantage of voice mail is that it grants freedom of movement. If you need to leave a message for a co-worker, you do not have to wait at a certain place for the answer. It will be in your mailbox when you are ready to listen. Voice mail is an excellent timesaving device. It cuts down significantly on the number of calls routed through beepers. In order to get the full use of this technology, you must check your messages several times a day.

The Office

When all of these alternatives have been tried, and there is still no way to leave a message or receive an answer, think "office." It is a central place where responses can be received and communication established. There is always someone there to take messages. If the message concerns a physician's order, the supervisor or charge nurse can be informed and receive the order for you if you are out seeing patients and are unable to receive the response yourself.

TIME MANAGEMENT

Patient time, documentation time, care coordination time, and travel time are the four components of a home care field day. To some extent, each one can be managed to produce maximum efficiency and effectiveness. Caseloads vary in size and also fluctuate from day to day. The number of admissions, discharges, deaths, and interrupted service due to rehospitalization are just a few of the factors influencing the number of patients in a caseload at any one time. Independent practice being the nature of home care, you are your own manager and can control each component of each day. Emergencies do happen. There are days when an exacerbation of congestive heart failure, a new form to use, or even a traffic jam can change a well-planned day into a nightmare. Fortunately, most days can be executed as planned.

Throughout the chapters in Part Two, *Home Care Nursing Practice,* suggestions have been made on how to handle specific difficulties. The following section examines each component of a day's work and how it can best be organized. Better time management helps both to improve output and to increase satisfaction with the day's accomplishments.

Patient Time

This is the actual time spent at patients' homes. On each admission to home care services, a plan of care is developed. Needs are identified; so are the outcomes to be achieved. Often, after the first visit, you will have a sense of how easily patient and caregivers will be able to grasp the points of your teaching, as well as how long treatments are going to take. This knowledge will assist in determining the length of each future visit.

1. Before each visit, know what you will concentrate on that particular day. You will have reviewed the chart at the office; review it again in your car just before entering the home. This procedure applies also if your agency uses "critical pathways," tools for identification of tasks or teaching to be done at each visit, scheduled over a pre-determined period of time.

> Derived from a term in computer technology, the critical pathway identifies a particular progression of events that include physician orders and standards of nursing practice. Each step in the pathway process must be completed in sequence before one proceeds to the next step. A deviation is a variance or detour from the pathway, which increases the period allotted to achieve specific goals (Harris, 1994, pp. 309–310).

The aim is maximum quality for minimum cost.

2. When in the home, concentrate on preidentified issues first. Then, handle new problems only if they need immediate attention. Determine if their resolution can wait until your next visit, after you have planned the time for them.

3. When teaching, use visual techniques to reinforce your instructions. This method can save a lot of time while enhancing the patient's memory.

4. While still in the home, write down, and prioritize, what needs to be done at the next visit. Most progress notes forms have a section at the end for this purpose.

Documentation Time

Also called "paperwork time," this will consume a large part of your day. As seen in Chapter 4, *Documentation,* there are several ways to do much work while still in the home. However, the concept of paperwork is not limited to patient progress notes. It applies to all pieces of writing, whether triggered by patient care, by reimbursement regulations, or necessary communications with the team members. By carefully planning the activities related to documentation, you should be able to remove some of the negative connotation often associated with home care paperwork.

1. Do as much charting as you can in the patient's home. If not possible, chart in your car, immediately after the visit. If the area is unsafe, move away, then chart.
2. Complete each day's progress notes that day. It is one of the most effective single factors in controlling that elusive time element.
3. Concise charting is a skill. Train yourself to describe problems and interventions without unnecessary articles or prepositions. Use abbreviations approved by your agency.
4. Keep an up-to-date calendar. Show due dates for 62-day recertifications of care plans and for Home Health Aide supervision, if appropriate, for each one of your patients.
5. Use checklist-type forms for review of systems on admission visits. If your agency does not have one already, develop your own. It is a valuable timesaving tool.

Care Coordination Time

As seen at the beginning of Chapter 5, care coordination is one of the most important responsibilities in caseload management. It is an integral part of patient and documentation time. It is performed wherever and whenever the actual needs require it. The treatment plan established on admission directs your actions. As a result, the time spent coordinating the care is fragmented. How can it then be done effectively without compromising outcomes?

When in patients' homes, handle each issue as it arises. Do as many telephone calls as possible from each home as the questions come up. For example, to the scheduler: Why did the home health aide not show up as scheduled today? To the supplies company: When is the commode being delivered? To the laboratory: What is the result of the Digoxin level drawn this morning? Utilize beepers and voice mail. Dealing with each issue immediately prevents accumulating the questions in the hope of finding more time at the end of the day's visits. Immediate action also has a positive impact on the patients, who are more likely to feel that somebody really cares about them as individuals.

Travel Time

The organization of a home care office reflects the districts of the city or area it serves. The divisions are determined by each agency, usually to accommodate travel time for field staff. They can be based on zip codes, density of population, or patient acuity. Depending on the size of the territory to be covered, there can be multiple districts, reflected in the number of teams or units in an office.

Travel time is easier to control if all or most of your patients are located in the same district. Unfortunately, because admissions do not occur equally in every part of town, it is not always possible for an agency to distribute patients evenly. Lots of effort goes into assignments, because supervisors are very aware of the impact travel time has on productivity. To decrease mileage:

1. Plan your visit schedule on different days of the week, to accommodate patients located in specific areas.
2. Keep maps in your car. Find the most direct route. (More on this subject can be found in Chapter 6: *Routes.*)

In-service classes, committee and staff meetings, and even blood pressure screening at various sites are other functions filling the home care nurse's day. Because of all these diverse activities, time management become even more crucial. Learning to utilize the office support staff effectively can ease some of the crunch. Assistance from the secretarial and administrative staff is particularly valuable for the new employee. When learning to plan your daily or monthly activities, consider asking for input from the office staff. They represent a wealth of information.

Even with the best of organization, there may be times when one becomes overwhelmed by the discrepancies between the time available in a day and all the things that need to be done. On those days, in order to catch up, it may be necessary to decrease the number of patients visited. Take that time to do whatever is called for to bring your care plans up to date. Some agencies allow an "office day" occasionally, to give case managers the opportunity to write recertifications (review of treatment plan every 62 days) and meet deadlines. Time management is a skill. Close attention to the fourfold time responsibilities of the case manager will make those catch-up days happen less and less frequently.

Chapter 6

PHYSICAL CHARACTERISTICS OF THE HOME CARE ENVIRONMENT

Knowing the environment facilitates effectiveness at work. The environment of a home care nurse is comprised of people's homes, the office, and the road. This section introduces the basic elements of each, and presents suggestions on how to handle some difficulties encountered during the course of a day's work.

A basic difference between home care and hospital work is the territory. In the hospital units, nurses are in charge, the patients being the guests. In home care, the reverse happens—nurses become the guests on the patient's turf. Consequently, no matter in what condition you find the house, apartment, room, or location, you must be respectful and nonjudgmental. While cultural differences influence the way people live, they should not distract you from your work.

PEOPLE'S HOMES

Ways To Gain Entry to Homes, with Permission, of Course

After receiving referrals from physicians, you set out to visit patients in their homes. It is not always as easy as it sounds. First you must be able to contact the patients; then you enter the homes. You become quickly aware of how many homes do not have telephones and how many doorbells are out of order. Other difficulties relate to patients. Many are bedbound, while still others are hard of hearing. Patients using wheelchairs, walkers, or crutches take time to get to the door, as do patients with chronic obstructive pulmonary diseases. They must all be given time to answer the doorbell.

Forgetfulness creates a problem of its own, especially when patients remember neither the appointment they just made nor the time of the visit. How can these obstacles be overcome so that you can legally enter patients' homes to carry out the doctor's orders?

If there are special requirements to either reach a patient or enter a home, these should be found on the registration sheet. Frequently, however, this information is missing. Here are a few suggestions if there are no telephone numbers listed for a patient:

1. Call the emergency phone number listed on the registration sheet and get all the information possible. The person answering may be willing to meet you or to have a friend or relative meet you at the patient's residence.
2. Call telephone information; the patient's telephone might have just been connected recently.
3. Call the hospital social worker or the discharge coordinator if one is listed on the registration sheet.
4. If unsuccessful with all of the above, go to the address.

If you are able to make contact with someone there, make arrangements for future visits:

1. Check if there is a telephone there or nearby and record the number.
2. Depending on agency policy, a duplicate key can perhaps be made for the visiting nurse. If so, it is important to reassure the patient that the key will remain with the chart and be strictly for the agency's use.
3. Arrangements often can be made with a neighbor, who will alert the patient of the nurse's visit that day.
4. Sometimes, patients prefer to drop their house key from a window after they hear the doorbell and identify the nurse.
5. If patients reside at a hotel with no telephone in the rooms, call the front desk and leave a message announcing the time of the visit.

If you reach a patient's home and the doorbell is out of order:

1. Ring the manager or neighbors, if in an apartment building. Apologize for disturbing them, explain the situation, and ask for entry.

2. Find a public phone nearby, call the patient, and explain the situation. The patient may come down and open the door, or ask a neighbor to do so.
3. Make suitable arrangements for subsequent visits.

In general, when reaching patients' homes, check the address carefully. Many people live in basement apartments or rooms located behind garages, which is not always obvious from the street. Some bedbound patients even operate their garage door opener from their beds to let nurses in. Try to gather as much information as possible over the telephone, if available, when making the first contact.

If patients are forgetful, remind them of your imminent visit by calling them from the previous patient's house. A telephone call from a street corner phone just prior to the visit can accomplish the same thing. If available, a cellular phone is an ideal solution when used at the patient's doorway. The idea is to prevent frightening them and also to make sure that they open the door for the visit.

There are many ways of gaining entry to homes as long as arrangements are made in advance. In some neighborhoods, the patients become very creative to protect their security. Whatever the means of entrance, make note of it in a very visible manner on the front of the chart. Follow the same procedure for patients who take time getting to the door. Patients and substitute nurses will thank you for the help. It will both save them valuable time and prevent frustration.

Bugs and Pets

During home visits, you will encounter fleas and multiple types of bugs. Pests are not selective; they can be found in any household and any neighborhood. Fleas manifest their presence only by ankle bites and itching, unless the home is so badly infested that the offenders are actually visible. Roaches and other insects can be seen crawling on the walls or over the furniture. At times, it is even difficult to find a suitable place to put the nursing bag. One cannot change the home environment in these cases, but if such problems are known before the visit, there are ways to protect against them to some extent.

Insect Repellents

A variety can be found at hardware or sports stores. Applied to the uncovered parts of the body, they protect against bites for up to approximately 10 hours.

"Miraculous Insecticide Chalk®"

Found in variety stores, this product is highly effective against fleas. A circle is drawn with the chalk at the inside bottom of the person's slacks to prevent pests from going any further. It remains effective until the garment is washed. It is harmless to humans or animals.

Flea bites and unexplained rashes are a constant threat, due to exposure to a variety of insects and the lack of hygiene in some homes. Most rashes disappear without treatment. If they persist, see a dermatologist.

Pets provide companionship to the elderly. They are usually very protective of their owners; consequently, they can be threatening to nurses at times. Another problem can be that they interfere with treatments. Cats have been seen jumping on beds when dressings were being changed. Others have leaped into or sprayed nursing bags. Dogs that can not be walked by their sick and frail owners often view the premises as a bathroom. This can be unsafe for owners, as well as nurses, who can easily slip when walking without looking at their feet. What can be done to keep animals at bay when making a visit, without offending the owner?

If the animal is threatening, ask the owner to place the dog in another room for the duration of the visit. Even if the dog is only barking, the same request can be made, so that the noise does not interfere with the conversation and the teaching process. Most people will comply if the demand is seen as reasonable.

No animals should be allowed on beds when dressings are being changed. Maintaining asepsis in some homes is difficult enough without fur or fleas contributing to contamination. Again, request that the cat or dog be put outside or in an adjacent room, if possible. Do not attempt to do this yourself; the most docile animal can turn aggressive if it feels that its master is being threatened.

Safety of the elderly can be compromised by small animals running through a room. An unsteady patient using a cane or a walker can be tripped. Warn patients to look carefully where they step when there is an animal around. Falls are traumatic, and even more so if caused by a favorite pet.

TVs, Telephones

Televisions are mentioned here because they can interfere with the effectiveness of your work. In many homes, televisions are on almost 24 hours a day. The constant noise becomes part of the background; people become oblivious to it. Only when they focus on the screen are they aware of the sound. For nurses who are trying to teach or listen to breath sounds, it makes concentration difficult. For patients, who may have a short attention span, in addition to being hard of hearing, it compromises the benefits of the instruction.

Another difficulty associated with TV is the influence of television on the scheduling of visits. Some patients are reluctant to miss favorite programs. You might need to work your schedule around it. Not very pleasant or practical, but a problem in home care's real world.

If the TV is too loud, ask politely that it be turned down. My experience is that most people will turn it off automatically, at your request. They understand the need to decrease distractions so they can hear the instructions provided. If you sense some reluctance, ask to use the "mute" control while leaving the picture on. It should be sufficient to complete a lung assessment and yet not be interpreted by the patient as too controlling.

A telephone is a basic convenience found in most homes. It can become a lifeline in an emergency, when you need to call a doctor or an ambulance from a home. Problems arise because many instruments are disconnected, for example, because bills have not been paid. Cordless telephones are sometimes inoperable because of failure to recharge the battery or because they have been dropped too many times.

Rotary, instead of touch tone telephones, present a special problem when you need to page somebody immediately; rotary telephones do not interface with beepers. What should you do in these cases, or when there is no phone?

1. If a physician needs to be contacted in an urgent situation, and there is no telephone, it will be up to you to find the nearest one. It could be at a neighbor's apartment or at the home next door. Pharmacies and corner stores are often willing to offer their telephones in dire emergencies. It helps to mention that "It is for your neighbor, Ms./Mr. at such and such address." Again, politeness is necessary, because you are on other people's territory.

2. If there is an immediate need to page a physician or a co-worker and there is no touchtone telephone, call the office. Explain the urgency of the situation and have the secretary page the person needed. Give the phone number of the patient so the return call can reach you quickly. Then wait. If there is no immediate answer, repeat the process. Physicians can also be paged in hospitals, especially before noon.

Home care nurses often must rely on relatives, friends, or neighbors to make contact with their patients. It is important, therefore, to gather as many phone numbers as possible, so that contact can be made and care be provided as soon as possible after the physician's referral.

Relatives and Friends

Without the assistance of relatives and friends, nurses could not effectively provide care in homes. For example, if a dressing must be changed twice a day, the nurse will do the morning treatment and teach the in-home helper to change the afternoon dressing. This team effort both facilitates the patient's recovery and gives the family a sense of participation.

At times, however, well-meaning relatives and friends may want an approach different from that ordered by the physician. They can be seen as very challenging and threatening to nurses new to the field. My experience is that these difficult people are usually the ones who most need reassurance and teaching. Many relatives respond positively if more time is spent explaining the disease process and discussing the goals to be achieved.

In some cases, they may remain antagonistic towards health care professionals. In this case, the nurse needs to inform the physician of the difficulty and follow that physician's recommendations. A visit by a different nurse the following day might work.

In general, it is worth the effort trying to develop a good relationship with relatives and friends so that patients can better benefit from teaching and treatment. Most people who come on strong when nurses visit their homes mean well. They have just gone through a traumatic time with their loved ones and thus may be overly protective. They might also have had a bad experience at the hospital, with the service, the nurses, or even the food or TV set. If that is the case, you will certainly hear about it. Do not take it personally. Listen to the complaints, discuss them with a supervisor, see if they are within the realm of home care nurses to correct, and act accordingly.

In more serious cases, it may be appropriate to call in a social worker. It is always helpful to have somebody else's point of view when it comes to such difficulties. Social workers deal with psychosocial aspects of family interaction and can provide useful insights into intricate situations. Learning how not to lose control under attack is a most useful skill in home care, where difficult situations are likely to develop when you least expect it.

Nurse's Safety

Safety is an important issue in home care, as elsewhere. Nurses are called on to provide care in all kinds of neighborhoods, increasing their vulnerability to the possibility of attack. Vigilance is necessary, no matter which district is covered, even the ones considered safe. Crime is an equal-opportunity provider. No neighborhoods are completely safe these days.

The "home" of home care covers a broad range of dwellings: single-family houses, apartments, hotel rooms, and even homeless shelters. Thus, the home care nurse needs to be extremely cautious when approaching an unfamiliar address. If there are people loitering nearby and the situation feels unsafe, it probably is. Call your supervisor rather than put yourself at risk. You will not be blamed for being cautious. Call your patient and the physician; explain the situation. If your agency has security guards, the visit can be rescheduled for the following day, with an escort.

Here are some general safety tips when working in the field:

1. Visit high-risk areas early in the day. Less activity in the streets means less risk of confrontation.
2. Familiarize yourself with the locations of the police and fire stations of your assigned district.
3. Plan your daily route carefully, to minimize driving through areas considered unsafe.
4. Keep the car doors locked at all times, both when driving and when charting in your car. Be especially alert at intersections, particularly when waiting for the light to change; carjacking, which is an armed vehicle theft, is a crime on the rise.
5. Make sure your car is in good working condition. It is a good idea to keep a spare key in your pocket. Attached to a credit card-sized piece of plastic, a spare key is available free to AAA members. Consider adding a whistle and a penlight to your key ring.
6. Park as close as possible to the home you are visiting, in a well-lighted area.
7. Consider adding a security device to your steering wheel, when parked.
8. If riding an elevator alone: "Stand near the control panel. If accosted, press all buttons. If a suspicious person enters the elevator, exit before the door closes" (San Francisco Police Department, 1993).
9. "Convenient and necessary as they are, pay phones can leave a woman (and man) vulnerable to attack. Don't stand with your head buried in the booth. Rather, stand at an angle to see if someone approaches, and be ready to get away if you have to (Safety experts advise the same posture at an automatic teller machine)" ("Personal vigilance," 1992).
10. Be sure someone at the office knows your schedule. If you must deviate from it, inform the office.

What indicates an unsafe home?

1. Illegal drug paraphernalia in evidence.

2. Weapons openly placed on the furniture or found in a bed with a patient.
3. Abusive language being used, escalating in intensity or directed at you.
4. When anyone is intoxicated.

It is then time to get out quickly, drive away, and report the incident to your supervisor. When weapons are found, each case should be evaluated individually. In these troubled times, many elderly patients are unwilling to let go of their weapons; they feel that it is their only protection.

Sexual Harassment

Sexual harassment can be described as "any unwelcome sexual advance, requests for favors, verbal or physical conduct of a sexual nature, or conduct on the job that creates an intimidating, hostile, or offensive working environment" (Thobaben, 1993, p. 66). In 1964, under Title VII of the Civil Rights Act, sex discrimination in the workplace was made illegal. However, the guidelines were defined only in the 1980s, by the Equal Employment Opportunities Commission.

No matter where nursing is practiced, uninvited sexual overtures are always a possibility. In home care, however, the nurse is generally alone in the patient's home. Potentially difficult situations can arise when least expected, and without witnesses. Patients' relatives could also be a source of problems at times. How can you protect yourself if you are sexually harassed?

1. Follow your agency's policy.
2. "Confront the harasser and clearly state that the attention is unwanted. Voice your displeasure directly to the harasser, repeatedly, if necessary" (ANA, 1993, pp. 2–3).
3. Keep a record of the incident: what, where, when, and was there any witness?
4. Contact your supervisor and report the situation.
5. Your agency will decide if it is safe for anyone to return or possibly discharge the patient, after informing the private physician.

The American Nurses Association provides detailed guidelines on sexual harassment, in their Workplace Information Series. See the Bibliography for more information.

Timing of Visits

What are the determining factors in scheduling visits to patients' homes? The number of patients seen in a day by a nurse varies. From 1–3 patients seen during the orientation, it reaches a productivity level of 5–8, based on agency standards and acuity.

Consequently, at first, there is more flexibility in scheduling patients. However, even at full productivity, many factors influencing timing remain the same. Being aware of them can save you valuable minutes throughout the day. Also, choosing the most appropriate time to visit patients will make them more receptive to your teaching. Here are some of the most common factors influencing visits:

1. *Purpose.* Calculate 30 minutes average duration for a standard visit (visit other than an admission or IV); 60–90 minutes for an admission.
2. *Address.* How far from the office does the patient live? How many patients to be seen in a day are located in the same part of town? Is it a designated escort area? Even if certain areas are not officially designated as low-safety areas, it may be better to visit in the morning, instead of the afternoon. Later, there may be more activity in the streets, and safety can be compromised. Check with your agency for its policy regarding escort areas.
3. *Language.* If a language other than English is spoken in the home, is there a family member available to interpret? Alternatively, a telephone translation service can be an excellent solution, if your agency chooses to subscribe. For example, the internationally available AT&T Language Line® offers an over-the-phone translation between English and 140 languages. Where language is a problem, you will want to add extra time to be sure your information is correctly understood.
4. *Treatments.* Treatments vary in length. For example: Foley catheter insertion, feeding tube instructions, or dressing changes for multiple wounds will all absorb more of your time. In cases of blood draw, choose the laboratory closest to the patient's home for delivery, insurance permitting.
5. *Other factors.* Frequently, nursing homes or other residential care facilities do not want their patients disturbed at mealtimes. Check with them about this issue when calling to make an appointment.

Patients' treatments (for example, dialysis, radiation therapy) at other facilities come first. Your visits need to be worked around them.

Some patients request not to be disturbed before a certain time, such as 10 a.m. After the first visit, you might be able to change this somewhat if you explain to the patient the importance of early visits (for example, blood glucose monitoring).

Lack of a telephone in a home or room can throw a schedule off, because you are never sure if the patient will be there (for example, in a Methadone program). On the other hand, these sometimes become the easiest visits to make because you can fit them in anytime at your convenience.

6. *Personal factors.* We should not underestimate the influence of personal factors on scheduling of visits. Some people function better in the morning, and others in the afternoon. Children might need to be taken to or picked up from schools. As long as the patients are well attended to, the productivity quotas met, and the paperwork handed in on time, you can usually organize your visits any way you want. It is another example of how flexible home care nursing can be.

People have their own routine. Many elderly patients also move slowly because of debilitating ailments. They will alter their routine to accommodate your visits because they realize the importance of these visits. Courtesy demands being on time. There will always be emergencies or events beyond our control. In these cases, a call from the previous home to the next patient to visit is in order.

After a few weeks of making home visits, you will sometimes amaze yourself at how precise your timing was in scheduling. Each visit took exactly the time you thought it would. Experience does pay off.

ON THE ROAD

Traffic: Survival, Safety

Driving is a constant source of stress, particularly in cities. There are fast drivers, always in a hurry, who pass left and right, without regard for the law. Couriers on bicycles weave in and out of traffic without giving signals. Detours, spills, torn-up streets, and traffic jams all add to the tension. As useful as cellular phones are, an animated conversation using one, while at the wheel, can be a source of distraction for an otherwise vigilant driver. I have also seen one driver, in heavy traffic, using his shaver, and a woman applying her makeup.

In addition to the stress faced by every driver, home care nurses have to deal with the pressure of finding the right address, a parking place, or a working telephone, several times a day, sometimes in unfamiliar neighborhoods. There are also other factors that can diminish their concentration at the wheel: lack of sleep because of a sick child at home, nervousness in anticipation of meeting a new patient, or the anxiety of not knowing how to handle a new home situation. Even the thought of seeing a very sick and dear patient once more can distract. As you become more experienced in the field, some of these stressors diminish. However, others are totally out of your control and must be dealt with. How then, do you survive the daily challenge of being at the wheel? Here are some practical suggestions for safety and survival:

1. *Drive within the speed limits.* Home care nurses are not exempt from the law.

> All states base their speed regulations on the Basic Speed Law: "No person shall drive a vehicle upon a highway at a speed greater than is reasonable or prudent having due regard for weather, visibility, the traffic on, and the surface and width of, the highway, and in no event at a speed which endangers the safety of persons or property" (California State Automobile Association, 1994).

The temptation to speed, especially if late for an appointment, is very strong at times. The added wear and tear is not worth it; one arrives at the location even more tense from having had to watch the traffic so intensely. Call the patient to be seen and let them know you are going to be late.

2. *Drive defensively.* The American Automobile Association (AAA) recommends managing time and space around the vehicle we are driving, so that seeing and being seen become priorities. At times, you might need to give up the right of way to avoid a potential accident. Being too forceful when another driver wants to push his way through is not worth the aggravation.

3. *Communicate your position to other drivers.* Use signal lights every time you make a move.

4. *Think safety.* After experiencing threatening situations in homes, such as finding yourself in the presence of substance abuse, or being confronted by a psychotic patient or family, the impulse to drive aimlessly for a while can be very strong. Resist this as much as you can. Drive to a close, safe area and park. Rest for a few minutes, and then drive back to the office where the difficult situation can be discussed with a supervisor. At a time like this, one is very vulnerable. Safe driving demands concentration.

A word of encouragement, after all of this, home care nurses have a very low rate of accidents. They do follow regulations and have good safety records in general.

Routes

After determining the addresses of the patients to be visited, the next step is finding the most direct route. There are many ways to get there. The one you want is the time- and stress-saver. Safety is also a major concern. Here are a few suggestions regarding choosing suitable routes:

1. Have on hand easy-to-read maps.
2. Concentrate on the main streets until you have become familiar with all parts of town. There are usually fewer stop signs on those streets, and the traffic flows better.
3. Drive along parks, small lakes or cemeteries; there are fewer intersections. Not having to watch both ways at all times for traffic eases stress.
4. Avoid, if possible, streets under repair, and long traffic signals. Especially at rush hour traffic, listen to the radio to keep informed of any traffic delay.

In general, choose the more direct routes to get there. Favor the more scenic ones after all the visits are completed. You deserve a break, and driving through pleasant surroundings can provide relaxation—not so much relaxation, however, that safety is compromised.

Parking

One major difficulty to be faced is parking. In cities already short of parking spaces, especially in downtown areas, the problem can be challenging. Minimizing time looking for suitable spots becomes very important. The "Visiting Nurse" sign placed conspicuously on the dashboard helps, but is not always a deterrent to a ticket. Expired meters or red zones are still illegal. Some cities are more lenient towards health care workers and give them a few minutes' reprieve if they are late getting back to their car. You should not take unnecessary chances. Parking tickets, which are neither reimbursable or deductible, can amount to a lot of money at the end of the year.

Home care gives nurses an opportunity to become proficient at parallel parking. There is a tendency for some people to go out of their way to avoid it. However, the maneuvers are easy to learn. It is definitely a time-saving skill, well worth learning. In addition, every day there are many occasions to practice when visiting patients.

1. The size of a car can make a lot of difference in how fast a parking place is located. The smaller the car, the easier the parking. Considering the fact that most parking is on the streets, this is not a factor to ignore. In addition, remember always to carry plenty of loose change to feed meters.
2. When calling patients to make appointments, ask if it is possible to park in their driveway. Unless they live in an apartment building, most

people are happy to oblige. Some, knowing how difficult it is to park in their area, even make the suggestion themselves. After seeing a patient for the first time, if there is some specific information about parking, make sure to write it down on the front of the chart. Other nurses, at subsequent visits, will thank you for the time you have saved them.

3. In certain parts of town, where parking places are most scarce, find your patient's location and then head for the parking garage closest to it. Optimism can be a time waster sometimes. After you have driven around the block a few times, there will never be any doubt in your mind about the course of action on your next visit.

Saving receipts from parking garages is important; they need to be handed in for reimbursement purposes.

Having to park a few blocks away from your destination might not always be a negative. Walking is very good exercise if you are wearing comfortable shoes. Of course, make sure the area is safe; be aware of the surroundings at all times.

PART III

APPENDIXES

A. Medicare Coverage of Services

B. Abbreviations

C. Educational Resources

D. Tools of the Trade

E. Your Car (As Transportation)
Your Car (As Office)
Your Car (As Classroom)

F. Occupational Hazards: Prevention

Appendix **A**

MEDICARE COVERAGE OF SERVICES

MEDICARE
COVERAGE OF SERVICES
Covered and Noncovered Home Health Services

203. CONDITIONS TO BE MET FOR COVERAGE OF HOME HEALTH SERVICES

Home health agency (HHA) services are covered by Medicare when the following criteria are met:

- The person to whom the services are provided is an eligible Medicare beneficiary.
- The HHA that is providing the services to the patient has in effect a valid agreement to participate in the Medicare program.
- The beneficiary qualifies for coverage of home health services as described in §204.
- The services for which payment is claimed are covered as described in §§205 and 206.
- Medicare is the appropriate payor.
- The services for which payment is claimed are not otherwise excluded from payment.

203.1 *Reasonable and Necessary Services*

A. *Background.*—In enacting the Medicare program, Congress recognized that the physician would play an important role in determining utilization of services. The law requires that payment can be made only if a physician certifies the need for services and establishes a plan of care. The Secretary is responsible for ensuring that the claimed services are covered by Medicare, including determining whether they are "reasonable and necessary."

B. *Determination of Coverage.*—The intermediary's decision on whether care is reasonable and necessary is based on information reflected in the home health plan of care (HCFA 485), in supplementary forms (e.g., HCFA 486 or an HHA's internal form), and the medical record concerning the unique medical condition of the individual patient. A coverage denial is not made solely on the basis of the reviewer's general inferences about patients with similar diagnoses or evidence regarding the patient's individual need for care. Additional information from the medical record must be requested when medical information needed to support a decision is not clearly present. The following examples illustrate this statement.

Examples of cases in which development of the case is needed:

EXAMPLE 1: A plan of care provides for daily skilled nursing visits for care of a pressure sore, but the description of the pressure sore and the dressing which is contained on the form causes the reviewer to question why daily skilled care is needed. The intermediary would not reduce the number of visits but would either request additional information to support the need for daily care or would request the nursing notes to determine if the patient required daily skilled care.

EXAMPLE 2: A patient with a diagnosis of congestive heart failure (CHF) has been hospitalized for 5 days. Posthospital skilled nursing care is ordered 3 x wk x 62 days for skilled observation, teaching of diet, medication compliance and signs and symptoms of the disease. The documentation on the HCFA 485 and supplementary form shows that the patient has had CHF for 10 years with an exacerbation requiring recent hospitalization. The medications are not shown as changed or new. The clinical findings are contradictory. There is a possibility that this patient requires skilled observation and teaching although the documentation does not give a clear picture of the patient's needs. Therefore, the case would be developed further to determine if the criteria for coverage were met.

Examples of cases which would be denied without further development:

EXAMPLE 3: A plan of care calls for vitamin B12 injections 1 x mo x 62 days for a patient who has been discharged from the hospital following a recent hip fracture. The patient has generalized weakness but there is no diagnosis or clinical symptoms shown to support

Medicare coverage of skilled nursing care for B12 injections. The claim would be denied without further development.

EXAMPLE 4: A patient has a primary diagnosis of back sprain that resulted in a 7-day hospitalization. The patient also has a secondary diagnosis of emphysema with an onset 2 years prior to the start of care. Following the hospitalization, the physician ordered skilled nursing 2 x wk x 4 weeks for skilled observation of vital signs and response to medication and aide services 2 x wk x 4 weeks for personal care. The documentation on the HCFA 485 and supplementary form shows that the patient is up as tolerated, able to walk 10 feet without resting and able to perform ADLs. Clinical facts show normal vital signs, with no reference to emphysema. The patient is on colace 100 mg BID. The documentation clearly does not support the medical necessity for skilled nursing care and the claim for the services would be denied without development.

Examples of cases in which payment may be made without further development:

EXAMPLE 5: A patient with a diagnosis of CHF has been hospitalized for five days. Post-hospital skilled nursing care is ordered 3 x wk x 60 days for skilled observation, teaching of a new diet regimen, compliance with multiple new medications, and signs and symptoms of the disease state. The documentation on the HCFA 485 and supplementary form shows the patient has had an acute exacerbation of a pre-existing CHF condition that required the recent acute hospitalization. The beneficiary is discharged from the hospital with a medication regimen changed from previous medications. The HCFA forms documenting the clinical evidence of the recent acute exacerbation of the beneficiary's cardiac condition combined with changed medications support the physician's order for care. Payment may be made without further development.

EXAMPLE 6: A plan of care provides for physical therapy treatments 3 x wk x 45 days for a patient who has been discharged from the hospital following a recent hip fracture. The patient was discharged using a walker 7 days before the start of home care. The HCFA form 485 and supplementary form show that the patient was discharged from the hospital with restricted mobility in ambulation, transfers, and climbing of stairs. The patient had an unsafe gait indicating a need for gait training and had not been instructed in stair climbing and a home exercise program. The goal of the physical therapy was to increase strength, range of motion and to progress from walker to cane with safe gait. Information on the relevant HCFA forms also indicates that the patient had a previous functional capacity of full ambulation, mobility, and self care. The claim may be paid without further development, since there are no objective clinical factors in the medical evidence to contradict the order of the patient's treating physician.

203.2 *Impact of Other Available Caregivers and Other Available Coverage on Medicare Coverage of Home Health Services.*—Where the Medicare criteria for coverage of home health services are met, patients are entitled by law to coverage of reasonable and necessary home health services.

Therefore, a patient is entitled to have the costs of reasonable and necessary services reimbursed by Medicare without regard to whether there is someone available to furnish them. However, where a family member or other person is or will be providing services that adequately meet the patient's needs, it would not be reasonable and necessary for HHA personnel to furnish such services. Ordinarily it can be presumed that there is no able and willing person to provide the services being rendered by the HHA unless the patient or family indicates otherwise, and objects to the provision of the services by the HHA, or the HHA has first hand knowledge to the contrary.

EXAMPLE: A beneficiary, who lives with an adult daughter and otherwise qualifies for Medicare coverage of home health services, requires the assistance of a home health aide for bathing and assistance with an exercise program to improve endurance. The daughter is unwilling to bathe her elderly father and assist him with the exercise program. Home health aide services to provide these services would be reasonable and necessary.

Similarly, a patient is entitled to have the costs of reasonable and necessary home health services reimbursed by Medicare even if the patient would qualify for institutional care (e.g., hospital care or skilled nursing facility care).

EXAMPLE: A patient who is being discharged from a hospital with a diagnosis of osteomyelitis and who requires continuation of the IV antibiotic therapy that was begun in the hospital was found to meet the criteria for Medicare coverage of skilled nursing facility services. If the patient also meets the qualifying criteria for coverage of home health services, payment may be made for the reasonable and necessary home health services the patient needs, notwithstanding the availability of coverage in a skilled nursing facility.

Medicare payment should be made for reasonable and necessary home health services where the patient is also receiving supplemental services that do not meet Medicare's definition of skilled nursing care or home health aide services.

EXAMPLE: A patient who needs skilled nursing care on an intermittent basis also hires a licensed practical (vocational) nurse to provide nighttime assistance while family members sleep. The care provided by the nurse, as respite to the family members, does not require the skills of a licensed nurse as defined in §205.1 and, therefore, has no impact on the patient's eligibility for Medicare payment of home health services even though another third party insurer may pay for that nursing care.

203.3 *Use of Utilization Screens and "Rules of Thumb"*.—Medicare recognizes that determinations of whether home health services are reasonable and necessary must be based on an assessment of each patient's individual care needs. Therefore, denial of services based on numerical utilization screens, diagnostic screens, diagnosis or specific treatment norms is not appropriate.

204. CONDITIONS THE PATIENT MUST MEET TO QUALIFY FOR COVERAGE OF HOME HEALTH SERVICES

To qualify for Medicare coverage of any home health services, the patient must meet each of the criteria specified in this section. Patients who meet each of these criteria are eligible to have payment made on their behalf for services which are discussed in §205 and §206.

204.1 *Confined to the Home.*—

A. *Patient Confined to the Home.*—In order for a patient to be eligible to receive covered home health services under both Part A and Part B, the law requires that a physician certify in all cases that the patient is confined to his/her home. (See §240.1.) An individual does not have to be bedridden to be considered as confined to the home. However, the condition of these patients should be such that there exists a normal inability to leave home and, consequently, leaving their homes would require a considerable and taxing effort. If the patient does in fact leave the home, the patient may nevertheless be considered homebound if the absences from the home are infrequent or for periods of relatively short duration, or are attributable to the need to receive medical treatment. Absences attributable to the need to receive medical treatment include attendance at adult day centers to receive medical care, ongoing receipt of outpatient kidney dialysis, and the receipt of outpatient chemotherapy or radiation therapy. It is expected that in most instances absences from the home that occur will be for the purpose of receiving medical treatment. However, occasional absences from the home for nonmedical purposes, e.g., an occasional trip to the barber, a walk around the block or a drive, would not necessitate a finding that the patient is not homebound if the absences are undertaken on an infrequent basis or are of relatively short duration and do not indicate that the patient has the capacity to obtain the health care provided outside rather than in the home.

Generally speaking, a patient will be considered to be homebound if he/she has a condition due to an illness or injury which restricts his/her ability to leave his/her place of residence except with the aid of supportive devices such as crutches, canes, wheelchairs, and walkers, the use of special transportation, or the assistance of another person or if leaving home is medically contraindicated. Some examples of homebound patients that illustrate the factors used to determine whether a homebound condition exists would be: (1) a patient paralyzed from a stroke who is confined to a wheelchair or who requires the aid of crutches in order to walk; (2) a patient who is blind or senile and requires the assistance of another person in leaving his/her residence; (3) a patient who has lost the use of his/her upper extremities and, therefore, is unable to open doors, use handrails on stairways, etc., and requires the assistance of another individual to leave his/her residence; (4) a patient who has just returned from a hospital stay involving surgery suffering from resultant weakness and pain and, therefore, his/her actions may be restricted by his/her physician to certain specified and limited activities such as getting out of bed only for a specified period of time, walking stairs only once a day, etc.; and (5) a patient with arteriosclerotic heart disease of such severity that he/she must avoid all stress and physical activity; and (6) a patient with a psychiatric problem if the illness is manifested in part by a refusal to leave home or is of such a nature that it would not be considered safe to leave home unattended, even if he/she has no physical limitations.

The aged person who does not often travel from home because of feebleness and insecurity brought on by advanced age would not be considered confined to the home for purposes of receiving home health services unless he/she meets one of the above conditions. A patient who requires skilled care must also be determined to be confined to the home in order for home health services to be covered.

Although a patient must be confined to the home to be eligible for covered home health services, some services cannot be provided at the patient's residence because equipment is required which cannot be made available there. If the services required by a patient involve the use of such equipment, the HHA may make arrangements with a hospital, skilled nursing facility, or a rehabilitation center to provide these services on an outpatient basis. (See §§200.2 and 206.5.) However, even in these situations, for the services to be covered as home health services the patient must be considered confined to his/her home; and to receive such outpatient services a homebound patient will generally require the use of supportive devices, special transportation, or the assistance of another person to travel to the appropriate facility.

If a question is raised as to whether a patient is confined to the home, the HHA will be asked to furnish the intermediary with the information necessary to establish that the patient is homebound as defined above.

B. *Patient's Place of Residence.*—A patient's residence is wherever he/she makes his/her home. This may be his/her own dwelling, an apartment, a relative's home, a home for the aged, or some other type of institution. However, an institution may not be considered a patient's home if the institution meets the requirements of §§1861(e) (1) or 1819(a) (1) of the Act. Included in this group are hospitals and skilled nursing facilities, as well as most nursing facilities under Medicaid

Thus, if a patient is in an institution or distinct part of an institution identified above, the patient is not entitled to have payment made for home health services under either Part A or Part B since these institutions may not be considered his/her residence. When a patient remains in a participating SNF following his/her discharge from active care, the facility may not be considered his/her residence for purposes of home health coverage.

204.2 *Services Are Provided Under a Plan of Care Established and Approved by a Physician.*—

A. *Content of the Plan of Care.*—The plan of care must contain all pertinent diagnoses, including the patient's mental status, the types of services, supplies, and equipment ordered, the frequency of the visits to be made, prognosis, rehabilitation potential, functional limitations, activities permitted, nutritional requirements, all medications and treatments, safety measures to protect against injury, instructions for timely discharge or referral, and any additional items the HHA or physician choose to include.

NOTE: This manual uses the term "plan of care" to refer to the medical treatment plan established by the treating physician with the assistance of the home health care nurse. Although HCFA previously used the term "plan of treatment," the Omnibus Budget Reconciliation Act of 1987 replaced that term with "plan of care" without a change in definition. HCFA anticipates that a discipline-oriented plan of care will be established, where appropriate, by an HHA nurse regarding nursing and home health aide services and by skilled therapists regarding specific therapy treatment. These plans of care may be incorporated within the physician's plan of care or separately prepared.

B. *Specificity of Orders.*—The orders on the plan of care must specify the type of services to be provided to the patient, both with respect to the professional who will provide them and the nature of the individual services, as well as the frequency of the services.

EXAMPLE: SN x 7/wk x 1 wk; 3/wk x 4 wk x 3 wk, (skilled nursing visits 7 times per week for 1 week; three times per week for 4 weeks; and two times per week ± for 3 weeks) for skilled observation and evaluation of the surgical site, for teaching sterile dressing changes and to perform sterile dressing changes. The sterile change consists of . . . (detail of procedure).

Orders for care may indicate a specific range in the frequency of visits to ensure that the most appropriate level of service is provided to home health patients. When a range of visits is ordered, the upper limit of the range is considered the specific frequency.

EXAMPLE: SN x 2–4/wk., x 4 wk; 1–2/wk x 4 wk for skilled observation and evaluation of the surgical site. . . .

Orders for services to be furnished "as needed" or "PRN" must be accompanied by a description of the patient's medical signs and symptoms that would occasion a visit and a specific limit on the number of those visits to be made under the order before an additional physician order would have to be obtained.

C. *Who Signs the Plan of Care.*—The physician who signs the plan of care must be qualified to sign the physician certification as described in 42 CFR 424.22.

D. *Timeliness of Signature.*—The plan of care must be signed before the bill is submitted to the intermediary for payment.

E. *Use of Oral (Verbal) Orders.*—When services are furnished based on a physician's oral order, the orders may be accepted and put in writing by personnel authorized to do so by applicable State and Federal laws and regulations, as well as by the HHA's internal policies. The orders must be signed and dated with the date of receipt by the registered nurse or qualified therapist (i.e., physical therapist, speech-language pathologist, occupational therapist, or medical social worker) responsible for furnishing or supervising the ordered services. The orders may be signed by the supervising registered nurse or qualified therapist after the services have been rendered, as long as HHA personnel who receive the oral orders notify that nurse or therapist before the service is rendered. Thus, the rendering of a service that is based on an oral order would not be delayed pending signature of the supervising nurse or therapist. Oral orders must be countersigned and dated by the physician before the HHA bills for the care in the same way as the plan of care.

EXAMPLE: The HHA acquires a verbal order for venipuncture for a patient to be performed on August 1. The HHA provides the venipuncture on August 1 and evaluates the patient's need for continued care. The physician signs the plan of care for the venipuncture on August 15. Since the HHA had acquired a verbal order prior to the delivery of services, the visit is considered to be provided under a plan of care established and approved by the physician.

Services which are provided in the subsequent certification period are considered to be provided under the subsequent plan of care where there is an oral order before the services provided in the subsequent period are furnished and the order is reflected in the medical record. However, services that are provided after the expiration of a plan of care, but before the acquisition of an oral order or a signed plan of care, cannot be considered to be provided under a plan of care.

EXAMPLE 1: The patient is under a plan of care in which the physician orders venipuncture every 2 weeks. The last day covered by the initial plan of care is July 31. The patient's next venipuncture is scheduled for August 5th, and the physician signs the plan of treatment for the new period on August 1st. The venipuncture on August 5th was provided under a plan of care established and approved by the physician.

EXAMPLE 2: The patient is under a plan of care in which the physician orders venipuncture every 2 weeks. The last day covered by the plan of care is July 31. The patient's next venipuncture is scheduled for August 5th, and the physician does not sign the plan of care until August 6th. The HHA acquires an oral order for the venipuncture before the August 5th visit, and therefore the visit is considered to be provided under a plan of care established and approved by the physician.

EXAMPLE 3: The patient is under a plan of care in which the physician orders venipuncture every 2 weeks. The last day covered by the plan of care is July 31. The patient's next venipuncture is scheduled for August 5th, and the physician does not sign the plan of care until August 6th. The HHA *does not* acquire a verbal order for the venipuncture before the August 5th visit, and therefore the visit cannot be considered to be provided under a plan of care established and approved by the physician. The prior plan of care expired and neither an oral order nor a signed plan of care was in effect on the date of the service. The visit is not covered.

Any increase in the frequency of services or addition of new services during a certification period must be authorized by a physician by way of a written or oral order prior to the provision of the increased or additional services.

F. *Periodic Review of the Plan of Care.*—The plan of care must be reviewed and signed by the physician who established the plan of care, in consultation with HHA professional personnel, at least every 62 days. Each review of a patient's plan of care must contain the signature of the physician and the date of review.

G. *Facsimile Signatures.*—The plan of care or oral order may be transmitted by facsimile machine. The HHA is not required to have the original signature on file. However, the HHA is responsible for obtaining original signatures if an issue surfaces that would require verification of an original signature.

H. *Alternative Signatures.*—HHAs that maintain patient records by computer rather than hard copy may use electronic signatures. However, all such entries must be appropriately authenticated and dated. Authentication must include signatures, written initials, or computer secure entry by a unique identifier of a primary author who has reviewed and approved the entry. The HHA must have safeguards to prevent unauthorized access to the records and a process for reconstruction of the records in the event of a system breakdown.

I. *Termination of the Plan of Care.*—The plan of care is considered to be terminated if the patient does not receive at least one covered skilled nursing, physical therapy, speech-language pathology service, or occupational therapy visit in a 62-day period unless the physician documents that the interval without such care is appropriate to the treatment of the patient's illness or injury.

204.3 *Under the Care of a Physician.*—The patient must be under the care of a physician who is qualified to sign the physician certification and plan of care in accord with 42 CFR 424.22.

A patient is expected to be under the care of the physician who signs the plan of care and the physician certification. It is expected, but not required for coverage, that the physician who signs the plan of care will see the patient, but there is no specified interval of time within which the patient must be seen.

204.4 *Needs Skilled Nursing Care on an Intermittent Basis, or Physical Therapy or Speech-Language Pathology Services or has Continued Need for Occupational Therapy.*—The patient must need one of the following types of skilled services:

- Skilled nursing care that:
  — Is reasonable and necessary as defined in §205.1 A and B, and
  — Is needed on an "intermittent" basis as defined in §205.1C, or
- Physical therapy as defined in §205.2A and B, or
- Speech-language pathology services as defined in §205.2A and C, or
- Have a continuing need for occupational therapy as defined in §205.2A and D.

The patient has a continued need for occupational therapy when:

- The services that the patient requires meet the definition of "occupational therapy" services of §205.2A and D, and
- The patient's eligibility for home health services has been established by virtue of a prior need for skilled nursing care, speech-language pathology services, or physical therapy in the current or prior certification period.

EXAMPLE: A patient who is recovering from a cerebral vascular accident has an initial plan of care that called for physical therapy, speech-language pathology services, and home health aide services. In the next certification period, the physician orders only occupational therapy and home health aide services because the patient no longer needs the skills of a physical therapist or a speech-language pathologist, but needs the services provided by the occupational therapist. The patient's need for occupational therapy qualifies him or her for home health services, including home health aide services (presuming that all other qualifying criteria are met).

204.5 *Physician Certification.*—The HHA must be acting upon a physician certification which is part of the plan of care (HCFA 485) and meets the requirements of this section for HHA services to be covered.

A. *Content of the Physician Certification.*—The physician must certify that:

1. The home health services are or were needed because the patient is or was confined to his/her home as defined in §204.1;
2. The patient needs or needed skilled nursing services on an intermittent basis or physical therapy or speech-language pathology services, or continues or continued to need occupational therapy after the need for skilled nursing care or physical therapy or speech-language pathology services ceased;
3. A plan of care has been established and is periodically reviewed by a physician; and
4. The services are or were furnished while the individual is or was under the care of a physician.

B. *Periodic Recertification.*—The physician certification may cover a period less than but not greater than 62 days (2 months).

C. *Who May Sign the Certification.*—The physician who signs the certification must be permitted to do so by 42 CFR 424.22.

205. COVERAGE OF SERVICES WHICH ESTABLISH HOME HEALTH ELIGIBILITY

For any home health services to be covered by Medicare, the patient must meet the qualifying criteria as specified in §204, including having a need for skilled nursing care on an intermittent basis, physical therapy, speech-language pathology services, or a continuing need for occupational therapy as defined in this section.

205.1 *Skilled Nursing Care.*—To be covered as skilled nursing services, the services must require the skills of a registered nurse or a licensed practical (vocational) nurse under the supervision of a registered nurse, must be reasonable and necessary to the treatment of the patient's illness or injury as discussed in §205.1A and B, and must be intermittent as discussed in §205.1C

A. *General Principles Governing Reasonable and Necessary Skilled Nursing Care.*—

1. A skilled nursing service is a service which must be provided by a registered nurse, or a licensed practical (vocational) nurse under the supervision of a registered nurse, to be safe and effective. In determining whether a service requires the skills of a nurse, consider both the inherent complexity of the service, the condition of the patient and accepted standards of medical and nursing practice.

Some services may be classified as a skilled nursing service on the basis of complexity alone, e.g., intravenous and intramuscular injections or insertion of catheters, and if reasonable and necessary to the treatment of the patient's illness or injury, would be covered on that basis. However, in some cases the condition of the patient may cause a service that would ordinarily be considered unskilled to be considered a skilled nursing service. This would occur when the patient's condition is such that the service can be safely and effectively provided only by a skilled nurse.

EXAMPLE 1: The presence of a plaster cast on an extremity generally does not indicate a need for skilled care. However, the patient with a pre-existing peripheral vascular or circulatory condition might need skilled nursing care to observe for complications, monitor medication administration for pain control and teach proper skin care to preserve skin integrity and prevent breakdown.

EXAMPLE 2: The condition of a patient who has irritable bowel syndrome, or who is recovering from rectal surgery, may be such that he/she can be given an enema safely and effectively only by a licensed nurse. If the enema is necessary to treat the illness or injury, the visit would be covered as a skilled nursing visit.

2. A service is not considered a skilled nursing service merely because it is performed by or under the direct supervision of a licensed nurse. Where a service can be safely and effectively performed (or self-administered) by the average nonmedical person without the direct supervision of a nurse, the service cannot be regarded as a skilled nursing service although a nurse actually provides the service. Similarly, the unavailability of a competent person to provide a nonskilled service, notwithstanding the importance of the service to the patient, does not make it a skilled service when the skilled nurse provides it.

EXAMPLE 1: Giving a bath does not ordinarily require the skills of a nurse and therefore would not be covered as a skilled nursing service unless the patient's condition is such that the bath could be given safely and effectively only by a nurse (as discussed in §205.1A.1. above).

EXAMPLE 2: A patient with a well-established colostomy absent complications may require assistance changing the colostomy bag because he/she cannot do it himself/herself and there is no one else to change the bag. Notwithstanding the need for the routine colostomy care, the care does not become a skilled nursing service when it is provided by the nurse.

3. A service which, by its nature, requires the skills of a licensed nurse to be provided safely and effectively continues to be a skilled service even if it is taught to the patient, the patient's family or other caregivers. Where the patient needs skilled nursing care and there is no one trained, able and willing to provide it, the services of a skilled nurse would be reasonable and necessary to the treatment of the illness or injury.

EXAMPLE: A patient was discharged from the hospital with an open draining wound which requires irrigation, packing and dressing twice each day. The HHA has taught the family to perform the dressing changes. The home health agency continues to see the patient for the wound care that is needed during the time that the family is not available and willing to provide the dressing changes. The wound care continues to be skilled nursing care, notwithstanding that the family provides it part of the time, and may be covered as long as it is required by the patient.

4. The skilled nursing service must be reasonable and necessary to the diagnosis and treatment of the patient's illness or injury within the context of the patient's unique medical condition. To be considered reasonable and necessary for the diagnosis or treatment of the patient's illness or injury, the services must be consistent with the nature and severity of the illness or injury, his or her particular medical needs, and accepted standards of medical and nursing practice. A patient's overall medical condition is a valid factor in deciding whether skilled services are needed. A patient's diagnosis should never be the sole factor in deciding that a service the patient needs is either skilled or unskilled.

The determination of whether the services are reasonable and necessary should be made in consideration that a physician has determined that the services ordered are reasonable and necessary. The services must, therefore, be viewed from the perspective of the condition of the patient when the services were ordered and what was, at that time, reasonably expected to be appropriate treatment for the illness or injury throughout the certification period.

EXAMPLE 1: A physician has ordered skilled nursing visits for a patient with a hairline fracture of the hip. In the absence of any underlying medical condition or illness, nursing visits would not be reasonable and necessary for treatment of the patient's hip injury.

EXAMPLE 2: A physician has ordered skilled nursing visits for injections of insulin and teaching of self-administration and self-management of the medication regimen for a patient with diabetes mellitus. Insulin has been shown to be a safe and effective treatment for diabetes mellitus, and therefore, the skilled nursing visits for the injections and the teaching of self-administration and management of the treatment regimen would be reasonable and necessary.

The determination of whether a patient needs skilled nursing care should be based solely upon the patient's unique condition and individual needs, without regard to whether the illness or injury is acute, chronic, terminal or expected to extend over a long period of time. In addition, skilled care may, dependent upon the unique condition of the patient, continue to be necessary for patients whose condition is stable.

EXAMPLE 1: Following a cerebral vascular accident (CVA), a patient has an in-dwelling Foley catheter because of urinary incontinence, and is expected to require the catheter for a long and indefinite period. Periodic visits to change the catheter as needed, to treat the symptoms of catheter malfunction and to teach proper patient care would be covered as long as they are reasonable and necessary, although the patient is stable and there is an expectation that the care will be needed for a long and indefinite period.

EXAMPLE 2: A patient with advanced multiple sclerosis undergoing an exacerbation of the illness needs skilled teaching of medications, measures to overcome urinary retention, and the establishment of a program designed to minimize the adverse impact of the exacerbation. The skilled nursing care the patient needs for a short period would be covered despite the chronic nature of the illness.

EXAMPLE 3: A patient with malignant melanoma is terminally ill, and requires skilled observation, assessment, teaching, and treatment. The patient has not elected coverage under Medicare's hospice benefit. The skilled nursing care that the patient requires would be covered, notwithstanding that his/her condition is terminal, because the services he needs require the skills of a nurse.

B. *Application of the Principles to Skilled Nursing Services.*—The following discussion of skilled nursing services applies the foregoing principles to specific skilled nursing services about which questions are most frequently raised.

1. *Observation and Assessment of Patient's Condition When Only the Specialized Skills of a Medical Professional Can Determine a Patient's Status.*—Observation and assessment of the patient's condition by a licensed nurse are reasonable and necessary skilled services when the likelihood of change

in a patient's condition requires skilled nursing personnel to identify and evaluate the patient's need for possible modification of treatment or initiation of additional medical procedures until the patient's treatment regimen is essentially stabilized. Where a patient was admitted to home health care for skilled observation because there was a reasonable potential of a complication or further acute episode, but did not develop a further acute episode or complication, the skilled observation services are still covered for 3 weeks or as long as there remains a reasonable potential for such a complication or further acute episode.

Information from the patient's medical history may support the likelihood of a future complication or acute episode and, therefore, may justify the need for continued skilled observation and assessment beyond the 3-week period. Moreover, such indications as abnormal/fluctuating vital signs, weight changes, edema, symptoms of drug toxicity, abnormal/fluctuating laboratory values, and respiratory changes on auscultation may justify skilled observation and assessment. Where these indications are such that it is likely that skilled observation and assessment by a nurse will result in changes to the treatment of the patient, then the services would be covered. There are cases where patients who are stable continue to require skilled observation and assessment (see example in §205.1 B. 13. d.). However, observation and assessment by a nurse is not reasonable and necessary to the treatment of the illness or injury where these indications are part of a longstanding pattern of the patient's condition, and there is no attempt to change the treatment to resolve them.

EXAMPLE 1: A patient with arteriosclerotic heart disease with congestive heart failure requires close observation by skilled nursing personnel for signs of decompensation, or adverse effects resulting from prescribed medication. Skilled observation is needed to determine whether the drug regimen should be modified or whether other therapeutic measures should be considered until the patient's treatment regimen is essentially stabilized.

EXAMPLE 2: A patient has undergone peripheral vascular disease treatment including a revascularization procedure (bypass). The incision area is showing signs of infection (e.g., heat, redness, swelling, drainage); patient has elevated body temperature. Skilled observation and monitoring of the vascular supply of the legs and the incision site is required until the signs of potential infection have abated and there is no longer a reasonable potential of infection.

EXAMPLE 3: A patient was hospitalized following a heart attack and, following treatment but before mobilization, is discharged home. Because it is not known whether exertion will exacerbate the heart disease, skilled observation is reasonable and necessary as mobilization is initiated until the patient's treatment regimen is essentially stabilized.

EXAMPLE 4: A frail 85 year old man was hospitalized for pneumonia. The infection was resolved, but the patient, who had previously maintained adequate nutrition, will not eat or eats poorly. The patient is discharged to the HHA for monitoring of fluid and nutrient intake, and assessment of the need for tube feeding. Observation and monitoring by licensed nurses of the patient's oral intake, output and hydration status is required to determine what further treatment or other intervention is needed.

EXAMPLE 5: A patient with glaucoma and a cardiac condition has a cataract extraction. Because of the interaction between the eye drops for the glaucoma and cataracts and the beta blocker for the cardiac condition, the patient is at risk for serious cardiac arrhythmias. Skilled observation and monitoring of the drug actions is reasonable and necessary until the patient's condition is stabilized.

EXAMPLE 6: A patient with hypertension suffered dizziness and weakness. The physician found that the blood pressure was too low and discontinued the hypertension medication. Skilled observation and monitoring of the patient's blood pressure is required until the blood pressure remains stable and in a safe range.

2. *Management and Evaluation of a Patient Care Plan.*—Skilled nursing visits for management and evaluation of the patient's care plan are also reasonable and necessary where underlying conditions or complications require that only a registered nurse can ensure that essential nonskilled care is achieving its purpose. For skilled nursing care to be reasonable and necessary for management and evaluation of the patient's plan of care, the complexity of the necessary unskilled services which are a necessary part of the medical treatment must require the involvement of licensed nurses to promote the patient's recovery and medical safety in view of the patient's overall condition.

EXAMPLE 1: An aged patient with a history of diabetes mellitus and angina pectoris is recovering from an open reduction of the neck of the femur. He requires among other services, careful skin care, appropriate oral medications, a diabetic diet, a therapeutic exercise program to preserve muscle tone and body condition, and observation to notice signs of deterioration in his/her condition or complications resulting from his/her restricted, but increasing mobility. Although any of the required services could be performed by a properly instructed person, that person would not have the capability to understand the relationship among the services and their effect on each other. Since the combination of the patient's condition, age and immobility create a high potential for patient's recovery and safety. The management of this plan of care requires skilled nursing personnel until the patient's treatment regimen is essentially stabilized.

EXAMPLE 2: An aged patient with a history of mild dementia is recovering from pneumonia which has been treated at home. The patient has had an increase in disorientation, has residual chest congestion, decreased appetite and has remained in bed, immobile, throughout the episode with pneumonia. While the residual chest congestion and recovery from pneumonia alone would not represent a high risk factor, the patient's immobility and increase in confusion could create a high probability of a relapse. In this situation, skilled oversight of the nonskilled services would be reasonable and necessary pending the elimination of the chest congestion and resolution of the persistent disorientation to ensure the patient's medical safety.

Where visits by a nurse are not needed to observe and assess the effects of the nonskilled services being provided to treat the illness or injury, skilled nursing care would not be considered reasonable and necessary to treat the illness or injury.

EXAMPLE: A physician orders one skilled nursing visit every 2 weeks and three home health aide visits each week for bathing and washing hair for a patient whose cerebral vascular accident has resulted in residual weakness on the left side. The cardiovascular condition is stable, and the patient has reached the maximum restoration potential. There are no underlying conditions which would necessitate the skilled supervision of a licensed nurse in assisting with bathing or hair washing. The skilled nursing visits are not necessary to manage and supervise the home health aide services and would not be covered.

3. *Teaching and Training Activities.*—Teaching and training activities which require skilled nursing personnel to teach a patient, the patient's family or caregivers how to manage his/her treatment regimen would constitute skilled nursing services. Where the teaching or training is reasonable and necessary to the treatment of the illness or injury, skilled nursing visits for teaching would be covered. The test of whether a nursing service is skilled relates to the skill required to teach and not to the nature of what is being taught. Therefore, where skilled nursing services

are necessary to teach an unskilled service, the teaching may be covered. Skilled nursing visits for teaching and training activities are reasonable and necessary where the teaching or training is appropriate to the patient's functional loss, illness or injury. Where it becomes apparent after a reasonable period of time that the patient, family or caregiver will not or is not able to learn or be trained, then further teaching and training would cease to be reasonable and necessary. The reason that the treatment was unsuccessful should be documented in the record. Notwithstanding that the teaching or training was unsuccessful, the services for teaching and training would be considered to be reasonable and necessary prior to the point that it became apparent that the teaching or training was unsuccessful, as long as such services were appropriate to the patient's illness, functional loss or injury.

EXAMPLE 1: A physician has ordered skilled nursing care for teaching a diabetic who has recently become insulin dependent. The physician has ordered teaching of self injection and management of insulin, signs and symptoms of insulin shock and actions to take in emergencies. The teaching services are reasonable and necessary to the treatment of the illness or injury.

EXAMPLE 2: A physician has ordered skilled nursing care to teach a patient to follow a new medication regimen (in which there is a significant probability of adverse drug reactions due to the nature of the drug and the patient's condition), signs and symptoms of adverse reactions to new medications and necessary dietary restrictions. After it becomes apparent that the patient remains unable to take the medications properly, cannot demonstrate awareness of potential adverse reactions, and is not following the necessary dietary restrictions, skilled nursing care for *further* teaching would not be reasonable and necessary.

EXAMPLE 3: A physician has ordered skilled nursing visits to teach self-administration of insulin to a patient who has been self injecting insulin for 10 years and there is no change in the patient's physical or mental status that would require reteaching. The skilled nursing visits would not be considered reasonable and necessary since the patient has a longstanding history of being able to perform the service.

EXAMPLE 4: A physician has ordered skilled nursing visits to teach self-administration of insulin to a patient who has been self-injecting insulin for 10 years because the patient has recently lost the use of the dominant hand and must be retrained to use the other hand. Skilled nursing visits to reteach self-administration of the insulin would be reasonable and necessary.

In determining the reasonable and necessary number of teaching and training visits, consideration must be given to whether the teaching and training provided constitute a reinforcement of teaching provided previously in an institutional setting or in the home or whether it represents the initial instruction. Where the teaching represents initial instruction, the complexity of the activity to be taught and the unique abilities of the patient are to be considered. Where the teaching constitutes a reinforcement, an analysis of the patient's retained knowledge and anticipated learning progress is necessary to determine the appropriate number of visits. Skills taught in a controlled institutional setting often need to be reinforced when the patient returns home. Where the patient needs reinforcement of the institutional teaching, additional teaching visits in the home are covered.

EXAMPLE 5: A patient recovering from pneumonia is being sent home requiring IV infusion of antibiotics 4 times per day. The patient's spouse has been shown how to administer the drug during the hospitalization and has been told the signs and symptoms of infection. The physician has also ordered home health services for a nurse to teach administration of the drug and the signs and symptoms requiring immediate medical attention. Teaching by the nurse in the home would be reasonable and necessary to continue that begun in the hospital, since the home environment, and the nature of the supplies used in the home, differ from that in the hospital.

Reteaching or retraining for an appropriate period may be considered reasonable and necessary where there is a change in the procedure or the patient's condition that requires reteaching, or where the patient, family or caregiver is not properly carrying out the task. The medical record should document the reason that the reteaching or retraining is required.

EXAMPLE 6: A well established diabetic who loses the use of his or her dominant hand would need to be retrained in self-administration of insulin.

EXAMPLE 7: A spouse who has been taught to perform a dressing change for a post surgical patient may need to be retaught wound care if the spouse demonstrates improper performance of wound care.

NOTE: There is no requirement that the patient, family or other caregiver be taught to provide a service if they cannot or choose not to provide the care.

Teaching and training activities which require the skills of a licensed nurse include, but *are not limited* to the following;

- Teaching the self-administration of injectable medications, or a complex range of medications;
- Teaching a newly diagnosed diabetic or caregiver all aspects of diabetes management, including how to prepare and to administer insulin injections, prepare and follow a diabetic diet, observe foot-care precautions, and observe for and understand signs of hyperglycemia and hypoglycemia;
- Teaching self-administration of medical gases;
- Teaching wound care where the complexity of the wound, the overall condition of the patient, or the ability of the caregiver makes teaching necessary;
- Teaching care for a recent ostomy or where reinforcement of ostomy care is needed;
- Teaching self-catheterization;
- Teaching self-administration of gastrostomy or enteral feedings;
- Teaching care for and maintenance of peripheral and central venous lines and administration of intravenous medications through such lines;
- Teaching bowel or bladder training when bowel or bladder dysfunction exists;
- Teaching how to perform the activities of daily living when the patient or caregiver must use special techniques and adaptive devices due to a loss of function;
- Teaching transfer techniques, e.g., from bed to chair, which are needed for safe transfer;
- Teaching proper body alignment and positioning, and turning techniques of a bed-bound patient;
- Teaching ambulation with prescribed assistive devices (such as crutches, walker, cane, etc.) that are needed due to a recent functional loss;
- Teaching prosthesis care and gait training;
- Teaching the use and care of braces, splints and orthotics and associated skin care;
- Teaching the proper care and application of any specialized dressings or skin treatments (for example, dressings or treatments needed by patients with severe or widespread fungal infections, active and severe psoriasis or eczema, or due to skin deterioration from radiation treatments);
- Teaching the preparation and maintenance of a therapeutic diet; and
- Teaching proper administration of oral medication, including signs of side-effects and avoidance of interaction with other medications and food.

4. *Administration of Medications.*—Although drugs and biologicals are specifically excluded from coverage by the statute (§1816(m)(5) of the Social Security Act), the services of a licensed nurse which are required to administer medications safely and effectively may be covered if they are reasonable and necessary to the treatment of the illness or injury.

a. Intravenous, intramuscular, or subcutaneous injections and infusions, and hypodermoclysis or intravenous feedings require the skills of a nurse to be performed (or taught) safely and effectively. Where these services are reasonable and necessary to treat the illness or injury, they may be covered. For these services to be reasonable and necessary, the medication being administered must be accepted as safe and effective treatment of the patient's illness or injury, and there must be a medical reason that the medication cannot be taken orally. Moreover, the frequency and duration of the administration of the medication must be within accepted standards of medical practice or there must be a valid explanation regarding the extenuating circumstances which justify the need for the additional injections.

(1) Vitamin B 12 injections are considered specific therapy only for the following conditions;
— Specified anemias: pernicious anemia, megaloblastic anemias, macrocytic anemias, fish tapeworm anemia,
— Specified gastrointestinal disorders; gastrectomy, malabsorption syndromes such as sprue and idiopathic steatorrhea, surgical and mechanical disorders such as resection of the small intestine, strictures, anastomosis and blind loop syndrome,
— Certain neuropathies; posteraloteral sclerosis, other neuropathies associated with pernicious anemia, during the acute phase or acute exacerbation of a neuropathy due to malnutrition and alcoholism.

For a patient with pernicious anemia caused by a B-12 deficiency, intramuscular or subcutaneous injection of vitamin B-12 at a dose of from 100 to 1000 micrograms no more frequently than once monthly is the accepted reasonable and necessary dosage schedule for maintenance treatment. More frequent injections would be appropriate in the initial or acute phase of the disease until it has been determined through laboratory tests that the patient can be sustained on a maintenance dose.

(2) *Insulin Injections.*—Insulin is customarily self-injected by patients or is injected by their families. However, where a patient is either physically or mentally unable to self-inject insulin and there is

no other person who is able and willing to inject the patient, the injections would be considered a reasonable and necessary skilled nursing service.

EXAMPLE: A patient who requires an injection of insulin once per day for treatment of diabetes mellitus, also has multiple sclerosis with loss of muscle control in the arms and hands, occasional tremors, and vision loss that causes inability to fill syringes or self inject insulin. If there is no able and willing caregiver to inject insulin, skilled nursing care would be reasonable and necessary for the injection of the insulin.

The prefilling of syringes with insulin (or other medication which is self-injected) does not require the skills of a licensed nurse, and therefore is not considered to be a skilled nursing service. If the patient needs someone only to prefill syringes (and therefore needs no skilled nursing care on an intermittent basis, or physical therapy or speech-language pathology services), the patient does not qualify for any Medicare coverage of home health care. Prefilling of syringes for self-administration of insulin or other medications is considered to be assistance with medications which are ordinarily self-administered and is an appropriate home health aide service. (See §206.1.) However, where State law requires that a nurse prefill syringes, a skilled nursing visit to prefill syringes is paid as a skilled nursing visit (if the patient otherwise needs skilled nursing care or physical therapy or speech-language pathology services), but is not considered to be a skilled nursing service.

b. *Oral Medications.*—The administration of oral medications by a nurse is not a reasonable and necessary skilled nursing care except in the specific situation in which the complexity of the patient's condition, the nature of the drugs prescribed and the number of drugs prescribed require the skills of a nurse to detect and evaluate side effects or reactions. The medical record must document the specific circumstances that cause administration of an oral medication to require skilled observation and assessment.
c. *Eye Drops and Topical Ointments.*—The administration of eye drops and topical ointments does not require the skills of a licensed nurse. Therefore, even if the administration of eyedrops or ointments is necessary to the treatment of an illness or injury, the patient cannot self-administer the drops, and there is no one available to administer them, the visits cannot be covered as a skilled nursing service. This section does not eliminate coverage for skilled nursing visits for observation and assessment of the patient's condition. (See §205.1.B.1.)

EXAMPLE 1: A physician has ordered skilled nursing visits to administer eye drops and ointments for a patient with glaucoma. The administration of eye drops and ointments does not require the skills of a nurse. Therefore, the skilled nursing visits cannot be covered as skilled nursing care, notwithstanding the importance of the administration of the drops as ordered.

EXAMPLE 2: A physician has ordered skilled nursing visits for a patient with a reddened area under the breast. The physician instructs the patient to wash, rinse, and dry the area daily and apply vitamin A and D ointment. Skilled nursing care is not needed to provide this treatment safely and effectively.

5. *Tube Feedings.*—Nasogastric tube, and percutaneous tube feedings (including gastrostomy and jejunostomy tubes), and replacement, adjustment, stabilization and suctioning of the tubes are skilled nursing services, and if the feedings are required to treat the patient's illness or injury, the feedings and replacement or adjustment of the tubes would be covered as skilled nursing services.

6. *Nasopharyngeal and Tracheostomy Aspiration.*—Nasopharyngeal and tracheostomy aspiration are skilled nursing services and, if required to treat the patient's illness or injury, would be covered as skilled nursing services.

7. *Catheters.*—Insertion and sterile irrigation and replacement of catheters, care of a suprapubic catheter, and in selected patients, urethral catheters, are considered to be skilled nursing services. Where the catheter is necessitated by a permanent or temporary loss of bladder control, skilled nursing services that are provided at a frequency appropriate to the type of catheter in use would be considered reasonable and necessary. Absent complications, Foley catheters generally require skilled care once approximately every 30 days and silicone catheters generally require skilled care once every 60–90 days and this frequency of service would be considered reasonable, and necessary. However, where there are complications that require more frequent skilled care related to the catheter, such care would, with adequate documentation, be covered.

EXAMPLE: A patient who has a Foley catheter due to loss of bladder control because of multiple sclerosis has a history of frequent plugging of the catheter and urinary tract infections. The physician has ordered skilled nursing visits once per month to change the catheter, and has left a "PRN" order for up to 3 additional visits per month for skilled observation and evaluation and/or catheter changes if the patient or family reports signs and symptoms of a urinary tract infection or a plugged catheter. During the certification period, the patient's family contacts the HHA because the patient has an elevated temperature, abdominal pain, and scant urine output. The nurse visits the patient and determines that the catheter is plugged and there are symptoms of a urinary tract infection. The nurse changes the catheter, and contacts the physician to advise him of her findings and to discuss treatment. The skilled nursing visit to change the catheter and to evaluate the patient would be reasonable and necessary to the treatment of the illness or injury.

8. *Wound Care.*—Care of wound, (including, but not limited to ulcers, burns, pressure sores, open surgical sites, fistulas, tube sites and tumor erosion sites) when the skills of a licensed nurse are needed to provide safely and effectively the services necessary to treat the illness or injury is considered to be a skilled nursing service. For skilled nursing care to be reasonable and necessary to treat a wound, the size, depth, nature of drainage (color, odor, consistency and quantity), condition and appearance of the skin surrounding the wound must be documented in the clinical findings so that an assessment of the need for skilled nursing care can be made. Coverage or denial of skilled nursing visits for wound care may not be based solely on the stage classification of the wound, but rather must be based on all of the documented clinical findings. Moreover, the plan of care must contain the specific instructions for the treatment of the wound. Where the physician has ordered appropriate active treatment (e.g. sterile or complex dressings, administration of prescription medications, etc.) of wounds with the following characteristics, the skills of a licensed nurse are usually reasonable and necessary:

a. Open wounds that are draining purulent or colored exudate or have a foul odor present or for which the patient is receiving antibiotic therapy;
b. Wounds with a drain or T-tube;
c. Wounds that require irrigation or instillation of a sterile cleansing or medicated solution into several layers of tissue and skin and/or packing with sterile gauze;
d. Recently débrided ulcers;
e. Pressure sores (decubitus ulcers) which present the following characteristics:

   - There is partial tissue loss with signs of infection such as foul odor or purulent drainage, or
   - There is full thickness tissue loss that involves exposure of fat or invasion of other tissue such as muscle or bone;

NOTE: Wound or ulcers that show redness, edema and induration, at times with epidermal blistering or desquamation do not ordinarily require skilled nursing care.

f. Wounds with exposed internal vessels or a mass which may have a proclivity for hemorrhage when a dressing is changed (e.g., post radical neck surgery, cancer of the vulva);
g. Open wounds or widespread skin complications following radiation therapy, or result from immune deficiencies or vascular insufficiencies;
h. Post-operative wounds where there are complications such as infection or allergic reaction or where there is an underlying disease that has a reasonable potential to adversely affect healing (e.g., diabetes);
i. Third degree burns, and second degree burns where the size of the burn or presence of complications causes skilled nursing care to be needed;
j. Skin conditions which require application of nitrogen mustard or other chemotherapeutic medication which present a significant risk to the patient; or
k. Other open or complex wounds that require treatment that can only be provided safely and effectively by a licensed nurse.

EXAMPLE 1: A patient has a second-degree burn with full thickness skin damage on his/her back. The wound is cleansed, followed by an application of Sulfamylon. While the wound requires skilled monitoring for signs and symptoms of infection or complications, the dressing change requires skilled nursing services.

EXAMPLE 2: A patient experiences a decubitus ulcer where the full thickness tissue loss extends through the dermis to involve subcutaneous tissue and the wound involves necrotic tissue. The physician's order is to apply a covering of a debriding ointment following vigorous irrigation. The wound is then packed loosely with wet to dry dressings or continuous moist dressing and covered with dry sterile gauze. Skilled nursing care is necessary for a proper treatment and understanding of cellular adherence and/or exudate or tissue healing or necrosis.

NOTE: This section relates to the direct, hands on skilled nursing care provided to patients with wounds, including any necessary dressing changes on those wounds. While a wound might not require this skilled nursing care, the wound may still require skilled monitoring for signs and symptoms of infection or complication (see §205.1.B.1) or skilled teaching of wound care to the patient or family (see §205.1.B.3)

9. *Ostomy Care.*—Ostomy care during the post-operative period and in the presence of associated complications where the need for skilled nursing care is clearly documented is a skilled nursing service. Teaching ostomy care remains skilled nursing care regardless of the presence of complications.

10. *Heat Treatments.*—Heat treatments which have been specifically ordered by a physician as part of active treatment of an illness or injury and require observation by a licensed nurse to adequately evaluate the patient's progress would be considered as skilled nursing services.

11. *Medical Gasses.*—Initial phases of a regimen involving the administration of medical gasses that are necessary to the treatment of the patient's illness or injury, would require skilled nursing care for skilled observation and evaluation of the patient's reaction to the gasses and to teach the patient and family when and how to properly manage the administration of the gasses.

12. *Rehabilitation Nursing.*—Rehabilitation nursing procedures, including the related teaching and adaptive aspects of nursing that are part of active treatment (e.g., the institution and supervision of bowel and bladder training programs) would constitute skilled nursing services.

13. *Venipuncture.*—Venipuncture when the collection of the specimen is necessary to the diagnosis and treatment of the patient's illness or injury and when the venipuncture cannot be performed in the course of regularly scheduled absences from the home to acquire medical treatment is a skilled nursing service. The frequency of visits for venipuncture must be reasonable within accepted standards of medical practice for treatment of the illness or injury.

For venipuncture to be reasonable and necessary:

— The physician order for the venipuncture for a laboratory test should be associated with a specific symptom or diagnosis, or the documentation should clarify the need for the test when it is not diagnosis/illness specific. In addition, the treatment must be recognized (in the *Physician's Desk Reference,* or other authoritative source) as being reasonable and necessary to the treatment of the illness or injury for venipunctures for monitoring the treatment to be reasonable and necessary.

— The frequency of testing should be consistent with accepted standards of medical practice for continued monitoring of a diagnosis, medical problem or treatment regimen. Even where the laboratory results are consistently stable, periodic venipuncture may be reasonable and necessary because of the nature of the treatment.

Examples of reasonable and necessary venipunctures for stabilized patients include, but are not limited to those described below. While these guidelines do not preclude a physician from ordering more frequent venipunctures for these laboratory tests, the HHA must present justifying documentation to support the reasonableness and necessity of more frequent testing.

a. Captopril may cause side effects such as leukopenia and agranulocytosis and it is standard medical practice to monitor the white blood cell count and differential count on a routine basis (every 3 months) when the results are stable and the patient is asymptomatic.
b. In monitoring phenytoin (e.g., Dilantin) administration, the difference between a therapeutic and a toxic level of phenytoin in the blood is very slight. Therefore, it is appropriate to monitor the level on a routine basis (every 3 months) when the results are stable and the patient is asymptomatic.
c. Venipuncture for fasting blood sugar (FBS):

   — An unstable insulin dependent or non-insulin dependent diabetic would require FBS more frequently than once per month if ordered by the physician.
   — Where there is a new diagnosis or where there has been a recent exacerbation, but the patient is not unstable, monitoring once per month would be reasonable and necessary.
   — A stable insulin or non-insulin dependent diabetic would require monitoring every 2–3 months.

d. Venipuncture for prothrombin

   — Where the documentation shows that the dosage is being adjusted, monitoring would be reasonable and necessary as ordered by the physician.
   — Where the results are stable within the therapeutic ranges, monthly monitoring would be reasonable and necessary.
   — Where the results are stable within non-therapeutic ranges, there must be documentation of other factors which would indicate why continued monitoring is reasonable and necessary.

EXAMPLE: A patient with coronary artery disease was hospitalized with atrial fibrillation and was subsequently discharged to the

HHA with orders for anticoagulation therapy. Monthly venipuncture as indicated is necessary to report prothrombin (protime) levels to the physician, notwithstanding that the patient's prothrombin time tests indicate essential stability.

14. *Student Nurse Visits.*—Visits made by a student nurse may be covered as skilled nursing care when an HHA participates in training programs that utilize student nurses enrolled in a school of nursing to perform skilled nursing services in a home setting. To be covered, the services must be reasonable and necessary skilled nursing care and must be performed under the general supervision of a registered or licensed nurse. The supervising nurse need not accompany the student nurse on each visit.

15. *Psychiatric Evaluation, Therapy, and Teaching.*—The evaluation, psychotherapy, and teaching activities needed by a patient suffering from a diagnosed psychiatric disorder require active treatment by a psychiatrically trained nurse and the costs of the psychiatric nurse's services may be covered as a skilled nursing care. Psychiatrically trained nurses are nurses who have special training and/or experience beyond the standard curriculum required for a registered nurse. The services of the psychiatric nurse are to be provided under a plan of care established and reviewed by a physician. A psychiatrist may also prescribe services of nonpsychiatric nursing such as intramuscular injections of behavior modifying medications.

Because the law precludes agencies that primarily provide care and treatment of mental diseases from participating as HHAs, psychiatric nursing must be furnished by an agency that does not primarily provide care and treatment of mental diseases. If a substantial number of an HHA's patients attend partial hospitalization programs or receive outpatient mental health services, the intermediary may verify whether the patients meet the eligibility requirements specified in §204 and whether the HHA is primarily engaged in care and treatment of mental diseases.

Services of a psychiatric nurse would not be considered reasonable and necessary to assess or monitor use of psychoactive drugs that are being used for nonpsychiatric diagnoses or to monitor the condition of a patient with a known psychiatric illness who is on treatment but is considered stable. A person on treatment would be considered stable if their symptoms were absent or minimal or if symptoms were present but were relatively stable and did not create a significant disruption in the patient's normal living situation.

EXAMPLE 1: A patient is homebound for medical conditions, but has a psychiatric condition for which he has been receiving medication. The patient's psychiatric condition has not required a change in medication or hospitalization for over 2 years. During a visit by the nurse, the patient's spouse indicates that the patient is awake and pacing most of the night and has begun ruminating about perceived failures in life. The nurse observes that the patient does not exhibit an appropriate level of hygiene and is dressed inappropriately for the season. The nurse comments to the patient about her observations and tries to solicit information about the patient's general medical condition and mental status. The nurse advises the physician about the patient's general medical condition and the new symptoms and changes in the patient's behavior. The physician orders the nurse to check blood levels of medication used to treat the patient's medical and psychiatric conditions. The physician then orders the psychiatric nursing service to evaluate the patient's mental health and communicate with the physician about whether additional intervention to deal with the patient's symptoms and behaviors is warranted.

EXAMPLE 2: A patient is homebound after discharge following hip replacement surgery and is receiving skilled therapy services for range of motion exercise and gait training. In the past, the patient had been diagnosed with clinical depression and was successfully stabilized on medication. There has been no change in her symptoms. The fact that the patient is taking an antidepressant does not indicate a need for psychiatric nursing services.

EXAMPLE 3: A patient was discharged after 2 weeks in a psychiatric hospital with a new diagnosis of major depression. The patient remains withdrawn, in bed most of the day, refusing to leave home. The patient has a depressed affect and continues to have thoughts of suicide, but is not considered to be suicidal. Psychiatric nursing is necessary for supportive interventions until antidepressant blood levels are reached and the suicidal thoughts are diminished further, to monitor suicide ideation, ensure medication compliance and patient safety, perform suicidal assessment, and teach crisis management and symptom management to family members.

C. *Intermittent Skilled Nursing Care.*—To meet the requirement for "intermittent" skilled nursing care, an individual must have a medically predictable recurring need for skilled nursing services. In most instances this definition will be met if a patient requires a skilled nursing service at least once every 60 days.

Since the need for "intermittent" skilled nursing care makes the individual eligible for other covered home health services, the intermediary should evaluate each claim involving skilled nursing services furnished less frequently than once every 60 days. In such cases, payment should be made only if documentation justifies a recurring need for reasonable, necessary, and medically predictable skilled nursing services. The following are examples of the need for infrequent, yet intermittent, skilled nursing services;

1. The patient with an indwelling *silicone* catheter who generally needs a catheter change only at 90-day intervals;
2. The person who experiences a fecal impaction (i.e., loss of bowel tone, restrictive mobility, and a breakdown in good health habits) and must be manually disimpacted. Although these impactions are likely to recur, it is not possible to pinpoint a specific timeframe; or
3. The blind diabetic who self-injects insulin may have a medically predictable recurring need for a skilled nursing visit at least every 90 days to observe and determine the need for changes in the level and type of care that have been prescribed, thus supplementing the physician's contacts with the patient.

Where the need for "intermittent" skilled nursing visits is medically predictable but a situation arises after the first visit making additional visits unnecessary, e.g., the patient is institutionalized or dies, the one visit would be reimbursable. However, a one-time order, e.g., to give gamma globulin following exposure to hepatitis, would not be considered a need for "intermittent" skilled nursing care since a recurrence of the problem which would require this service is not medically predictable.

Although most patients require services no more frequently than several times a week, Medicare will pay for part-time (as defined in §206.7) medically reasonable and necessary skilled nursing care 7 days a week for a *short* period of time (2–3 weeks). There may also be a few cases involving unusual circumstances where the patient's prognosis indicates a medical need for daily skilled services beyond 3 weeks. As soon as the patient's physician makes this judgment, which usually should be made before the end of the 3-week period, the home health agency must forward medical documentation justifying the need for such additional services and include an estimate of how much longer daily skilled services will be required.

A person expected to need more or less *full-time skilled nursing care over an extended period of time,* i.e., a patient who requires institutionalization, would usually not qualify for home health benefits.

205.2 *Skilled Therapy Services.—*

A. *General Principles Governing Reasonable and Necessary Physical Therapy, Speech-Language Pathology Services, and Occupational Therapy.—*

1. The service of a physical, speech-language pathologist or occupational therapist is a skilled therapy service if the inherent complexity of the service is such that it can be performed safely and/or effectively only by or under the general supervision of a skilled therapist. To be covered, the skilled services must also be reasonable and necessary to the treatment of the patient's illness or injury or to the restoration of maintenance of function affected by the patient's illness or injury. It is necessary to determine whether individual therapy services are skilled and whether, in view of the patient's overall condition, skilled management of the services provided is needed although many or all of the specific services needed to treat the illness or injury do not require the skills of a therapist.

2. The development, implementation management and evaluation of a patient care plan based on the physician's orders constitute skilled therapy services when, because of the patient's condition, those activities require the involvement of a skilled therapist to meet the patient's needs, promote recovery and ensure medical safety. Where the skills of a therapist are needed to manage and periodically reevaluate the appropriateness of a maintenance program because of an identified danger to the patient, such services would be covered even if the skills of a therapist are not needed to carry out the activities performed as part of the maintenance program.

3. While a patient's particular medical condition is a valid factor in deciding if skilled therapy services are needed, the diagnosis or prognosis should never be the sole factor in deciding that a service is or is not skilled. The key issue is whether the skills of a therapist are needed to treat the illness or injury, or whether the services can be carried out by nonskilled personnel.

4. A service that is ordinarily considered nonskilled could be considered a skilled therapy service in cases in which there is clear documentation that, because of special medical complications, skilled rehabilitation personnel are required to perform or supervise the service or to observe the patient. However, the importance of a particular service to a patient or the frequency with which it must be performed does not, by itself, make a nonskilled service into a skilled service.

5. The skilled therapy services must be reasonable and necessary to the treatment of the patient's illness or injury within the context of the patient's unique medical condition. To be considered reasonable and necessary for the treatment of the illness or injury;

a. The services must be consistent with the nature and severity of the illness or injury, the patient's particular medical needs, including the requirement that the amount, frequency and duration of the services must be reasonable,

b. The services must be considered, under accepted standards of medical practice, to be specific, safe, and effective treatment for the patient's condition, and
c. The services must be provided with the expectation, based on the assessment made by the physician of the patient's rehabilitation potential, that;

   - The condition of the patient will improve materially in a reasonable and generally predictable period of time, or
   - The services are necessary to the establishment of a safe and effective maintenance program.

Services involving activities for the general welfare of any patient, e.g., general exercises to promote overall fitness or flexibility and activities to provide diversion or general motivation, do not constitute skilled therapy. Those services can be performed by nonskilled individuals without the supervision of a therapist.

d. Services of skilled therapists for the purpose of teaching the patient, family or caregivers necessary techniques, exercises or precautions are covered to the extent that they are reasonable and necessary to treat illness or injury. However, visits made by skilled therapists to a patient's home solely to train other HHA staff (e.g., home health aides) are not billable as visits since the HHA is responsible for ensuring that its staff is properly trained to perform any service it furnishes. The cost of a skilled therapist's visit for the purpose of training HHA staff is an administrative cost to the agency.

EXAMPLE: A patient with a diagnosis of multiple sclerosis has recently been discharged from the hospital following an exacerbation of her condition which has left her wheelchair bound and, for the first time, without any expectation of achieving ambulation again. The physician has ordered physical therapy to select the proper wheelchair for her long term use, to teach safe use of the wheelchair and safe transfer techniques to the patient and family. Physical therapy would be reasonable and necessary to evaluate the patient's overall needs, to make the selection of the proper wheelchair and to teach the patient and family safe use of the wheelchair and proper transfer techniques.

e. The amount, frequency, and duration of the services must be reasonable.

B. *Application of the Principles to Physical Therapy Services.*—The following discussion of skilled physical therapy services applies the principles in §205.2A to specific physical therapy services about which questions are most frequently raised.

1. *Assessment.*—The skills of a physical therapist to assess a patient's rehabilitation needs and potential or to develop and/or implement a physical therapy program are covered when they are reasonable and necessary because of the patient's condition. Skilled rehabilitation services concurrent with the management of a patient's care plan include objective tests and measurements such as, but not limited to, range of motion, strength, balance coordination endurance or functional ability.

2. *Therapeutic Exercises.*—Therapeutic exercises which must be performed by or under the supervision of the qualified physical therapist to ensure the safety of the patient and the effectiveness of the treatment, due either to the type of exercise employed or to the condition of the patient, constitute skilled physical therapy.

3. *Gait Training.*—Gait evaluation and training furnished to a patient whose ability to walk has been impaired by neurological, muscular or skeletal abnormality require the skills of a qualified physical therapist and constitute skilled physical therapy and are considered reasonable and necessary if training can be expected to improve materially the patient's ability to walk.

Gait evaluation and training that is furnished to a patient whose ability to walk has been impaired by a condition other than a neurological, muscular or skeletal abnormality would nevertheless be covered where physical therapy is reasonable and necessary to restore the lost function.

EXAMPLE 1: A physician has ordered gait evaluation and training for a patient whose gait has been materially impaired by scar tissue resulting from burns. Physical therapy services to evaluate the patient's gait, establish a gait training program, and provide the skilled services necessary to implement the program would be covered.

EXAMPLE 2: A patient who has had a total hip replacement is ambulatory but demonstrates weakness, and is unable to climb stairs safely. Physical therapy would be reasonable and necessary to teach the patient to safely climb and descend stairs.

Repetitive exercises to improve gait, or to maintain strength and endurance and assistive walking are appropriately provided by nonskilled persons and ordinarily do not require the skills of a physical therapist. Where such services are performed by a physical therapist as part of the initial design and establishment of a safe and effective maintenance program, the services would, to the extent that they are reasonable and necessary, be covered.

EXAMPLE: A patient who has received gait training has reached his/her maximum restoration potential and the physical therapist is teaching the patient and family how to perform safely the activities that are a part of a maintenance program. The visits by the physical therapist to demonstrate and teach the activities (which by themselves do not require the skills of a therapist) would be covered since they are needed to establish the program.

4. *Range of Motion.*—Only a qualified physical therapist may perform range of motion tests and, therefore, such tests are skilled physical therapy.

Range of motion exercises constitute skilled physical therapy only if they are part of an active treatment for a specific disease state, illness, or injury, that has resulted in a loss or restriction of mobility (as evidenced by physical therapy notes showing the degree of motion lost and the degree to be restored). Range of motion exercises unrelated to the restoration of a specific loss of function often may be provided safely and effectively by nonskilled individuals. Passive exercises to maintain range of motion in paralyzed extremities that can be carried out by nonskilled persons do not constitute skilled physical therapy.

However, as indicated in section 205.2A4, where there is clear documentation that, because of special medical complications (e.g., susceptible to pathological bone fractures), the skills of a therapist are needed to provide services that ordinarily do not need the skills of a therapist, then the services would be covered.

5. *Maintenance Therapy.*—Where repetitive services that are required to maintain function involve the use of complex and sophisticated procedures, the judgement and skill of a physical therapist might be required for the safe and effective rendition of such services. If the judgment and skill of a physical therapist are required to treat the illness or injury safely and effectively, the services would be covered as physical therapy services.

EXAMPLE: Where there is an unhealed, unstable fracture that requires regular exercise to maintain function until the fracture heals, the skills of a physical therapist would be needed to ensure that the fractured extremity is maintained in proper position and alignment during maintenance range of motion exercises.

Establishment of a maintenance program is a skilled physical therapy service where the specialized knowledge and judgement of a qualified physical therapist is required for the program to be safely carried out and the treatment aims of the physician achieved.

EXAMPLE: A Parkinson's patient or a patient with rheumatoid arthritis who has not been under a restorative physical therapy program may require the services of a physical therapist to determine what type of exercises are required for the maintenance of his/her present level of function. The initial evaluation of the patient's needs, the designing of a maintenance program appropriate to the capacity and tolerance of the patient and the treatment objectives of the physician, the instruction of the patient, family or caregivers to carry out the program safely and effectively and such reevaluations as may be required by the patient's condition, would constitute skilled physical therapy.

While a patient is under a restorative physical therapy program, the physical therapist should regularly reevaluate his/her condition and adjust any exercise program the patient is expected to carry out himself or with the aid of supportive personnel to maintain the function being restored. Consequently, by the time it is determined that no further restoration is possible (i.e., by the end of the last restorative session) the physical therapist will already have designed the maintenance program required and instructed the patient or caregivers in carrying out the program.

6. *Ultrasound, Shortwave, and Microwave Diathermy Treatments.*—These treatments must always be performed by or under the supervision of a qualified physical therapist and are skilled therapy.

7. *Hot Packs, Infra-Red Treatments, Paraffin Baths and Whirlpool Baths.*—Heat treatments and baths of this type ordinarily do not require the skills of a qualified physical therapist. However, the skills, knowledge and judgment of a qualified physical therapist might be required in the giving of such treatments or baths in a particular case, e.g., where the patient's condition is complicated by circulatory deficiency, areas of desensitization, open wounds, fractures or other complications.

C. *Application of the General Principles to Speech-Language Pathology Services.*—Speech-language pathology services are those services necessary for the diagnosis and treatment of speech and language disorders that result in communication disabilities and for the diagnosis and treatment of swallowing disorders (dysphagia), regardless of the presence of a communication disability. The following discussion of skilled speech-language pathology services applies the principles to specific speech-language pathology services about which questions are most frequently raised.

1. The skills of a speech-language pathologist are required for the assessment of a patient's rehabilitation needs (including the causal factors and the severity of the speech and language disorders), and rehabilitation potential. Reevaluation would only be considered reasonable and necessary if the patient exhibited a change in functional speech or motivation, clearing of confusion or the remission of some other medical condition that previously contraindicated speech-language pathology services. Where a patient is undergoing restorative speech-language pathology services, routine reevaluations are considered to be a part of the therapy and could not be billed as a separate visit.

2. The services of a speech-language pathologist would be covered if they are needed as a result of an illness, or injury and are directed towards specific speech/voice production.

3. Speech-language pathology would be covered where the service can only be provided by a speech-language pathologist and where it is reasonably expected that the service will materially improve the patient's ability to independently carry out any one or a combination of communicative activities of daily living in a manner that is measurably at a higher level of attainment than that prior to the initiation of the services.

4. The services of a speech-language pathologist to establish a hierarchy of speech-voice-language communication tasks and cueing that directs a patient toward speech-language communication goals in the plan of care would be covered speech-language pathology services.

5. The services of a speech-language pathologist to train the patient, family, or other caregivers to augment the speech-language communication, treatment or to establish an effective maintenance program would be covered speech-language pathology services.

6. The services of a speech-language pathologist to assist patients with aphasia in rehabilitation of speech and language skills is covered when needed by a patient.

7. The services of a speech-language pathologist to assist patients with voice disorders to develop proper control of the vocal and respiratory systems for correct voice production are covered when needed by a patient.

D. *Application of the General Principles to Occupational Therapy.*—The following discussion of skilled occupational therapy services applies the principles to specific occupational therapy services about which questions are most frequently raised.

1. *Assessment*—The skills of an occupational therapist to assess and reassess a patient's rehabilitation needs and potential or to develop and/or implement an occupational therapy program are covered when they are reasonable and necessary because of the patient's condition.

2. *Planning, Implementing and Supervision of Therapeutic Programs.*—The planning, implementing and supervision of therapeutic programs including, but not limited to those listed below are skilled occupational therapy services, and if reasonable and necessary to the treatment of the patient's illness or injury would be covered.

a. Selecting and teaching task oriented therapeutic activities designed to restore physical function.

EXAMPLE: Use of woodworking activities on an inclined table to restore shoulder, elbow and wrist range of motion lost as a result of burns.

b. Planning, implementing and supervising therapeutic tasks and activities designed to restore sensory-integrative function.

EXAMPLE: Providing motor and tactile activities to increase sensory output and improve response for a stroke patient with functional loss resulting in a distorted body image.

c. Planning, implementing and supervising of individualized therapeutic activity programs as part of an overall "active treatment" program for a patient with a diagnosed psychiatric illness.

EXAMPLE: Use of sewing activities which require following a pattern to reduce confusion and restore reality orientation in a schizophrenic patient.

d. Teaching compensatory techniques to improve the level of independence in the activities of daily living.

EXAMPLE: Teaching a patient who has lost use of an arm how to pare potatoes and chop vegetables with one hand.

EXAMPLE: Teaching a stroke patient new techniques to enable him to perform feeding, dressing and other activities of daily living as independently as possible.

e. The designing, fabricating and fitting of orthotic and self-help devices.

EXAMPLE: Construction of a device which would enable an individual to hold a utensil and feed himself independently.

EXAMPLE: Construction of a hand splint for a patient with rheumatoid arthritis to maintain the hand in a functional position.

f. Vocational and prevocational assessment and training that is directed toward the restoration of function in the activities of daily living lost due to illness or injury would be covered. Where vocational or prevocational assessment and training is related solely to specific employment opportunities, work skills or work settings, such services would not be covered because they would not be directed toward the treatment of an illness or injury.

3. *Illustration of Covered Services.—*

EXAMPLE 1: A physician orders occupational therapy for a patient who is recovering from a fractured hip and who needs to be taught compensatory and safety techniques with regard to lower extremity dressing, hygiene, toileting and bathing. The occupational therapist will establish goals for the patient's rehabilitation (to be approved by the physician), and will undertake the teaching of the techniques necessary for the patient to reach the goals. Occupational therapy services would be covered at a duration and intensity appropriate to the severity of the impairment and the patient's response to treatment.

EXAMPLE 2: A physician has ordered occupational therapy for a patient who is recovering from a CVA. The patient has decreased range of motion, strength and sensation in both the upper and lower extremities on the right side and has perceptual and cognitive deficits resulting from the CVA. The patient's condition has resulted in decreased function in activities of daily living (specifically bathing, dressing, grooming, hygiene and toileting). The loss of function requires assistive devices to enable the patient to compensate for the loss of function and to maximize safety and independence. The patient also needs equipment such as himi-slings to prevent shoulder subluxation and a hand splint to prevent joint contracture and deformity in the right hand. The services of an occupational therapist would be necessary to assess the patient's needs, develop goals (to be approved by the physician), manufacture or adapt the needed equipment to the patient's use, teach compensatory techniques, strengthen the patient as necessary to permit use of compensatory techniques, and provide activities that are directed towards meeting the goals governing increased perceptual and cognitive function. Occupational therapy services would be covered at a duration and intensity appropriate to the severity of the impairment and the patient's response to treatment.

206. COVERAGE OF OTHER HOME HEALTH SERVICES

206.1 *Skilled Nursing Care, Physical Therapy, Speech-Language Pathology Services, and Occupational Therapy.*—Where the patient meets the qualifying criteria in §204, Medicare covers skilled nursing services that meet the requirements of §§205.1 A and B and §206.7, physical therapy that meets the requirements of §§205.2 A and B, speech-language pathology services that meet the requirements of §§205.2A and C, and occupational therapy that meets the requirements of §§205.2 A and D.

Home health coverage is not available for services furnished to a qualified patient who is no longer in need of one of the qualifying skilled services specified in §205. Therefore, dependent services furnished after the final qualifying skilled service are not covered, except when the dependent service was followed by a qualifying skilled service as a result of the unexpected inpatient admission or death of the patient or due to some other unanticipated event.

206.2 *Home Health Aide Services.*—For home health aide services to be covered, the patient must meet the qualifying criteria as specified in §204; the services provided by the home health aide must be part-time or intermittent as discussed in §206.7; the services must meet the definition of home health aide services of this section; and the services must be reasonable and necessary to the treatment of the patient's illness or injury.

The reason for the visits by the home health aide must be to provide hands-on personal care of the patient or services which are needed to maintain the patient's health or to facilitate treatment of the patient's illness or injury.

The physician's order should indicate the frequency of the home health aide services required by the patient. These services may include but are not limited to;

a. *Personal Care.*—Personal care means:

- Bathing, dressing, grooming, caring for hair, nail and oral hygiene that are needed to facilitate treatment or prevent deterioration of the patient's health, changing the bed linens of an incontinent patient, shaving, deodorant application, skin care with lotions and/or powder, foot care, and ear care.
- Feeding, assistance with elimination (including enemas unless the skills of a licensed nurse are required due to the patient's condition), routine catheter care and routine colostomy care, assistance with ambulation, changing position in bed, assistance with transfers.

EXAMPLE 1: A physician has ordered home health aide visits to assist the patient in personal care because the patient is recovering from a stroke and continues to have significant right side weakness which causes him to be unable to bathe, dress or perform hair and oral care. The plan of care established by the HHA nurse sets forth the specific tasks with which the patient needs assistance. Home health aide visits at an appropriate frequency would be reasonable and necessary to assist in these tasks.

EXAMPLE 2: A physician ordered four home health aide visits per week for personal care for a multiple sclerosis patient who is unable to perform these functions because of increasing debilitation. The home health aide gave the patient a bath twice per week and washed hair on the other two visits each week. Only two visits are reasonable and necessary since the services could have been provided in the course of two visits.

EXAMPLE 3: A physician ordered seven home health aide visits per week for personal care for a bed-bound, incontinent patient. All visits are reasonable and necessary because the patient has extensive personal care needs.

EXAMPLE 4: A patient with a well established colostomy forgets to change the bag regularly and has difficulty changing the bag. Home health aide services at an appropriate frequency to change the bag would be considered reasonable and necessary to the treatment of the illness or injury.

b. Simple dressing changes which do not require the skills of a licensed nurse.

EXAMPLE: A patient who is confined to the bed has developed a small reddened area on the buttocks. The physician has ordered home health aide visits for more frequent repositioning, bathing and the application of a topical ointment and a gauze 4 x 4. Home health aide visits at an appropriate frequency would be reasonable and necessary.

c. Assistance with medications that are ordinarily self-administered and which do not require the skills of a licensed nurse to be provided safely and effectively.

NOTE: Prefilling of insulin syringes is ordinarily performed by the diabetic as part of the self-administration of the insulin and, unlike the injection of the insulin, does not require the skill of a licensed nurse to be performed properly. Therefore, if the prefilling of insulin syringes is performed by HHA staff, it is considered to be a home health aide service. However, where State law precludes the provision of this service by other than a licensed nurse or physician, Medicare will make payment for this service, when covered, as though it were a skilled nursing service. Where the patient needs only prefilling of insulin syringes and does not need skilled nursing care on an intermittent basis, or physical therapy or speech-language pathology services or have a continuing need for occupational therapy, then Medicare cannot cover any home health services to the patient (even if State law requires that the insulin syringes be filled by a licensed nurse).

d. Assistance with activities which are directly supportive of skilled therapy services but do not require the skills of a therapist to be safely and effectively performed, such as routine maintenance exercises, and repetitive practice of functional communication skills to support speech-language pathology services.
e. Routine care of prosthetic and orthotic devices.

When a home health aide visits a patient to provide a health related service as discussed above, the home health aide may also perform some incidental services that do not meet the definition of a home health aide service (e.g., light cleaning, preparation of a meal, taking out the trash, shopping). However, the purpose of a home health aide visit may not be to provide these incidental services since they are not health related services, but rather are necessary household tasks that must be performed by anyone to maintain a home.

EXAMPLE 1: A home health aide visits a recovering stroke patient whose right side weakness and poor endurance cause her to be able to leave the bed and chair only with extreme difficulty. The physician has ordered physical therapy and speech-language pathology services for the patient and has ordered home health aide services three or four times per week for personal care, assistance with ambulation as mobility increases, and assistance with repetitive speech exercises as her impaired speech improves. The home health aide also provides incidental household services such as preparation of meals, light cleaning and taking out the trash. The patient lives with an elderly frail sister who is disabled and cannot perform either the personal care or the incidental tasks. The home health aide visits at a frequency appropriate to the performance of the health related services would be covered, notwithstanding the incidental provision of noncovered services (i.e., the household services) in the course of the visits.

EXAMPLE 2: A physician orders home health aide visits three times per week. The only services provided are light housecleaning, meal preparation and trash removal. The home health aide visits cannot be covered, notwithstanding their importance to the patient, because the services provided do not meet Medicare's definition of "home health aide services."

206.3 *Medical Social Services.*—Medical social services that are provided by a qualified medical social worker or a social work assistant under the supervision of a qualified medical social worker may be covered as home health services where the patient meets the qualifying criteria specified in §204, and:

- The services of these professionals are necessary to resolve social or emotional problems that are or are expected to be an impediment to the effective treatment of the patient's medical condition or his or her rate of recovery, and
- The plan of care indicates how the services that are required necessitate the skills of a qualified social worker or a social work assistant under the supervision of a qualified medical social worker to be performed safely and effectively.

Where both of these requirements for coverage are met, services of these professionals that may be covered include, but are not limited to:

- Assessment of the social and emotional factors related to the patient's illness, need for care, response to treatment and adjustment to care,
- Assessment of the relationship of the patient's medical and nursing requirements to the patient's home situation, financial resources and availability of community resources,
- Appropriate action to obtain available community resources to assist in resolving the patient's problem. (Note: Medicare does not cover the services of a medical social worker to complete or assist in the completion of an application for Medicaid because Federal regulations require the State to provide assistance in completing the application to anyone who chooses to apply for Medicaid);
- Counseling services which are required by the patient; and
- Medical social services furnished to the patient's family member or caregiver on a short-term basis when the HHA can demonstrate that a brief intervention (that is, two or three visits) by a medical social worker is necessary to remove a clear and direct impediment to the effective treatment of the patient's medical condition or to his or her rate of recovery. To be considered "clear and direct," the behavior or actions of the family member or caregiver must plainly obstruct, contravene, or prevent the patient's medical treatment or

rate of recovery. Medical social services to address general problems that do not clearly and directly impede treatment or recovery as well as long-term social services furnished to family members, such as ongoing alcohol counseling, are not covered.

NOTE: Participating in the development of the plan of treatment, preparing clinical and progress notes, participating in discharge planning and inservice programs, and acting as a consultant to other agency personnel are appropriate administrative costs to the HHA.

EXAMPLE 1: The physician has ordered a medical social worker assessment of a diabetic patient who has recently become insulin dependent and is not yet stabilized. The nurse, who is providing skilled observation and evaluation to try to restabilize the patient notices during her visits that supplies left in the home for the patient's use appear to be frequently missing, and that the patient is not compliant with the regimen and refuses to discuss the matter. The assessment by a medical social worker would be reasonable and necessary to determine if there are underlying social or emotional problems that are impeding the patient's treatment.

EXAMPLE 2: A physician has ordered an assessment by a medical social worker for a multiple sclerosis patient who is unable to move anything but her head and who has an indwelling catheter. The patient has experienced recurring urinary tract infections and multiple infected ulcers. The physician ordered medical social services after the HHA indicated to him that the home was not well cared for, and that the patient appeared to be neglected much of the time, and the relationship between the patient and family was very poor. The physician and HHA were concerned that social problems created by family caregivers were impeding the treatment of the recurring infections and ulcers. The assessment and follow-up for counseling both the patient and the family by a medical social worker would be reasonable and necessary.

EXAMPLE 3: A physician is aware that a patient with arteriosclerosis and hypertension is not taking medications as ordered and is not adhering to dietary restrictions because he is unable to afford the medication and is unable to cook. The physician orders several visits by a medical social worker to assist in resolving these problems. The visits by the medical social worker to review the patient's financial status, discuss options, and make appropriate contacts with social services agencies or other community resources to arrange for medications and meals would be a reasonable and necessary medical social service.

EXAMPLE 4: A physician has ordered counseling by a medical social worker for a patient with cirrhosis of the liver who has recently been discharged from a 28-day inpatient alcohol treatment program to her home that she shares with an alcoholic and neglectful adult child. The physician has ordered counseling several times a week to assist the patient in remaining free of alcohol and in dealing with the adult child. These services would be covered until the patient's social situation ceased to impact on her recovery and/or treatment.

EXAMPLE 5: A physician has ordered medical social services for a patient who is worried about her financial arrangements and payment for medical care. The services ordered are to arrange Medicaid if possible and resolve unpaid medical bills. There is no evidence that the patient's concerns are adversely impacting recovery or treatment of her illness or injury. Medical social services cannot be covered.

EXAMPLE 6: A physician has ordered medical social services for a patient of extremely limited income who has incurred large unpaid hospital and other medical bills following a significant illness. The patient's recovery is adversely affected because the patient is not maintaining a proper therapeutic diet, and cannot leave home to acquire the medication necessary to treat his/her illness. The medical social worker reviews the patient's financial status, arranges meal service to resolve the dietary problem, arranges for home delivered medications, gathers the information necessary for application to Medicaid to acquire coverage for the medications the patient needs, files the application on behalf of the patient, and follows up repeatedly with the Medicaid State agency.

The medical social services that are necessary to review the financial status of the patient, arrange for meal service, arrange for the medications to be delivered to the home, and arrange for the Medicaid State agency to assist the patient with the application for Medicaid are covered. The services related to the assistance in filing the application for Medicaid and the follow up on the application are not covered since they are provided by the State agency free of charge, and hence the patient has no obligation to pay for such assistance.

EXAMPLE 7: A physician has ordered medical social services for an insulin dependent diabetic whose blood sugar is elevated because she has run out of syringes and missed her insulin dose for two days. Upon making the assessment visit, the medical social worker learns that the patient's daughter, who is also an insulin dependent diabetic, has come to live with the patient because she is out of work. The daughter is now financially dependent on the patient for all of her financial needs and has been using the patient's insulin syringes. The social worker assesses the patient's financial resources and determines that they are adequate to support the patient and meet her own medical needs, but are not sufficient to support the daughter. She also counsels the daughter and helps her access community resources. These visits would be covered but only to the extent that the services are necessary to prevent interference with the patient's treatment plan.

EXAMPLE 8: An Alzheimer's patient is being cared for by his wife. The nurse learns that the wife has not been giving the patient his/her medication correctly and seems distracted and forgetful about various aspects of the patient's care. In a conversation with the nurse, the wife relates that she is feeling depressed and overwhelmed by the patient's illness. The nurse contacts the patient's physician who orders a social work evaluation. In her assessment visit, the social worker learns that the patient's wife is so distraught over her situation that she cannot provide adequate care to the patient and is interfering with the patient's treatment program. While there, the social worker counsels the wife and assists her with referrals to a support group and her private physician for evaluation of her depression.

EXAMPLE 9: The parent of a dependent disabled child has been discharged from the hospital following a hip replacement. Although arrangements for care of the disabled child during the hospitalization were made, the child has returned to the home. During a visit to the patient, the nurse observes that the patient is transferring the child from bed to a wheelchair. In an effort to avoid impeding the patient's recovery, the nurse contacts the patient's physician to order a visit by a social worker to mobilize family members or otherwise arrange for temporary care of the disabled child.

206.4 *Medical Supplies (Except for Drugs and Biologicals) and the Use of Durable Medical Equipment.*—

A. *Medical Supplies.*—Medical supplies are items that, due to their therapeutic or diagnostic characteristics, are essential in enabling HHA personnel to carry out effectively the care the physician has ordered for the treatment or diagnosis of the patient's illness or injury. Supplies fit into two categories. They are classified as:

- *Routine* because they are used in small quantities for patients during the usual course of most home visits; or

- *Nonroutine* because they are needed to treat a patient's specific illness or injury in accordance with the physician's plan of care and meet further conditions discussed in more detail below.

All HHAs are expected to separately identify in their records the cost of medical and surgical supplies that are not routinely furnished in conjunction with patient care visits and the use of which are directly identifiable to an individual patient.

1. *Routine Supplies (Nonbillable).*—Routine supplies are supplies that are customarily used during the course of most home care visits. They are usually included in the staff's supplies and not designated for a specific patient. These supplies are included in the cost per visit of home health care services. Routine supplies would not include those supplies that are specifically ordered by the physician or are essential to HHA personnel in order to effectuate the plan of care.

Examples of supplies which are usually considered routine include, but are not limited to:

- *Dressings and Skin Care*
  Swabs, alcohol preps, and skin prep pads
  Tape removal pads
  Cotton balls
  Adhesive and paper tape
  Non-sterile applicators
  4 x 4s
- *Infection Control Protection*
  Non-sterile gloves
  Aprons
  Masks
  Gowns
- *Blood Drawing Supplies*
  Specimen containers
- *Other*
  Thermometers
  Tongue depressors

There are occasions when the supplies listed in the above examples would be considered nonroutine and thus would be considered a billable supply, i.e., if they are required in quantity, for recurring need, and are included in the plan of care. Examples include, but are not limited to, tape and 4x4s for major dressings.

2. *Nonroutine Supplies (Billable)*—Nonroutine supplies are identified by the following conditions:

- The HHA follows a consistent charging practice for Medicare and non-Medicare patients receiving the item;
- The item is directly identifiable to an individual patient;
- The cost of the item can be identified and accumulated in a separate cost center; and
- The item is furnished at the direction of the patient's physician and is specifically identified in the plan of care.

All nonroutine supplies must be specifically ordered by the physician or the physician's order for services must require the use of the specific supplies to be effectively furnished.

The charge for nonroutine supplies is excluded from the per visit costs.

Examples of supplies which can be considered nonroutine include, but are not limited to:

- *Dressings/Wound Care*
  Sterile dressings
  Kling and Kerlix rolls
  Telfa pads
  Eye pads
  Sterile solutions, ointments
  Sterile applicators
  Sterile gloves
- *IV Supplies*
- *Ostomy Supplies*
- *Catheters and Catheter Supplies*
  Foley catheters
  Drainage bags, irrigation trays
- *Enemas and Douches*
- *Syringes and Needles*
- *Home Testing*
  Blood glucose monitoring strips
  Urine monitoring strips

Consider other items that are often used by persons who are not ill or injured to be medical supplies only where (1) the item is recognized as having the capacity to serve a therapeutic or diagnostic purpose in a specific situation, and (2) the item is required as a part of the actual physician-prescribed treatment of a patient's existing illness or injury. For example, items that generally serve a routine hygienic purpose, e.g., soaps and shampoos and items that generally serve as skin conditioners, e.g., baby lotion, baby oil, skin softeners, powders, lotions, are not considered medical supplies unless the particular item is recognized as serving a specific therapeutic purpose in the physician's prescribed treatment of the patient's existing skin (scalp) disease or injury.

Limited amounts of medical supplies may be left in the home between visits where repeated applications are required and rendered by the patient or other caregivers. These items must be part of the plan of care in which the home health staff are actively involved. For example, the patient is independent in insulin injections but the nurse visits once a day to change wound dressings. The wound dressings/irrigation solution may be left in the home between visits. Do not leave supplies such as needles, syringes, and catheters that require administration by a nurse in the home between visits.

D. *Durable Medical Equipment.*—Durable medical equipment which meets the requirements of §220 is covered under the home health benefit, with the patient responsible for payment of a 20 percent coinsurance.

206.5 *Services of Interns and Residents.*—Home health services include the medical services of interns and residents-in-training under an approved hospital teaching program if the services are ordered by the physician who is responsible for the plan of care and the HHA is affiliated with or is under common control of a hospital furnishing the medical services. Approved means:

A. Approved by the Accreditation Council for Graduate Medical Education;

B. In the case of an osteopathic hospital, approved by the Committee on Hospitals of the Bureau of Professional Education of the American Osteopathic Association;

C. In the case of an intern or resident-in-training in the field of dentistry, approved by the Council on Dental Education of the American Dental Association; or

D. In the case of an intern or resident-in-training in the field of podiatry, approved by the Council on Podiatric Education of the America Podiatric Association.

206.6 *Outpatient Services.*—Outpatient services include any of the items or services described above that are provided under arrangements on an outpatient basis at a hospital, skilled nursing facility (SNF), or rehabilitation center, and that (1) require equipment not readily available at the patient's place of residence, or (2) are furnished while the patient is at the facility to receive services. The hospital or SNF must be qualified providers of services. See §200.3 for special provisions for the use of the facilities of rehabilitation centers. The cost of transporting a patient to a facility cannot be paid.

206.7 *Part-time or Intermittent Home Health Aide and Skilled Nursing Services.—*

Where a patient qualifies for coverage of home health services, Medicare covers either part-time or intermittent home health aide services and skilled nursing services.

A. *Definition of Part-time.—*Part-time means any number of days per week:

- Up to and including 28 hours per week of skilled nursing and home health aide services combined for less than 8 hours per day; or
- Up to 35 hours of skilled nursing and home health aide services combined for less than 8 hours per day subject to review by fiscal intermediaries on a case by case basis, based upon documentation justifying the need for and reasonableness of such additional care.

B. *Definition of "Intermittent".—*"Intermittent" means:

- Up to and including 28 hours per week of skilled nursing and home health aide services combined provided on a less than daily basis;
- Up to 35 hours per week of skilled nursing and home health aide services combined which are provided on a less than daily basis, subject to review by fiscal intermediaries on a case by case basis, based upon documentation justifying the need for and reasonableness of such additional care; or
- Up to and including full-time (i.e., 8 hours per day) skilled nursing and home health aide services combined which are provided and needed 7 days per week for temporary, but not indefinite, periods of time of up to 21 days with allowances for extensions in exceptional circumstances where the need for care in excess of 21 days is finite and predictable.

C. *Impact on Care Provided in Excess of "Intermittent" or "Part-time" Care.—* Home health aide and/or skilled nursing care in excess of the amounts of care which meet these definitions of part time or intermittent may be provided to a home care patient or purchased by other payors without bearing on whether the home health aide and skilled nursing care meets the Medicare definitions of part time or intermittent.

EXAMPLE: A patient needs skilled nursing care monthly for a catheter change and the HHA also renders needed daily home health aide services 24 hours per day which will be needed for a long and indefinite period of time. The HHA bills Medicare for the skilled nursing and home health aide services which were provided before the 35th hour of service each week and bills the patient (or another payer) for the remainder of the care. If the intermediary determines that the 35 hours of care are reasonable and necessary, Medicare would therefore cover the 35 hours of skilled nursing and home health aide visits.

D. *Application of This Policy Revision.*—A patient must meet the longstanding and unchanged qualifying criteria for Medicare coverage of home health services, before this policy revision becomes applicable to skilled nursing services and/or home health aide services. The definition of "intermittent" with respect to the need for skilled nursing care where the patient qualifies for coverage based on the need for "skilled nursing care on an intermittent basis" remains unchanged. Specifically:

- This policy revision always applies to home health aide services when the patient qualifies for coverage;
- This policy revision applies to skilled nursing care only when the patient needs physical therapy or speech therapy or continued occupational therapy, and also needs skilled nursing care; and
- If the patient needs skilled nursing care but does not need physical therapy, speech-language pathology services or occupational therapy, the patient must still meet the longstanding and unchanged definition of "intermittent" skilled nursing care in order to qualify for coverage of any home health services.

Note. From U.S. Department of Health and Human Services, Health Care Financing Administration. Medicare program home health agency. (April 1996). *Health insurance manual–11*, transmittal revision No. 277, section 203–206.6 inclusively. Washington, DC: Government Printing Office.

Appendix **B**

ABBREVIATIONS

ADL	Activities of Daily Living
AIDS	Acquired Immunodeficiency Syndrome
ANA	American Nurses Association
CDC	Centers for Disease Control and Prevention
CEO	Chief Executive Officer
CFO	Chief Financial Officer
CHAP	Community Health Accreditation Program
COO	Chief Operating Officer
CQI	Continuous Quality Improvement
CVO	Confirmation of Verbal Order
DME	Durable Medical Equipment
DNR	Do Not Resuscitate
DRG	Diagnostic-Related Group
FI	Fiscal Intermediary
HCA	Home Care Aide
HCFA	Health Care Financing Administration
HHA	Home Health Agency
HHA	Home Health Aide
HHAAA	Homemaker-Home Aide Association of America
HIM–11	Health Insurance Manual–11
HIV	Human Immunodeficiency Virus
HMO	Health Maintenance Organization
IV	Intravenous
JCAHO	Joint Commission on Accreditation of Healthcare Organizations

(continued)

Abbreviations *(continued)*

LPN	Licensed Practical Nurse
LVN	Licensed Vocational Nurse
MSW	Medical Social Worker
NAHC	National Association for Home Care
NLN	National League for Nursing
OSHA	Occupational Safety and Health Administration
OT	Occupational Therapy
PCA	Personal Care Aide
PT	Physical Therapy
PTA	Physical Therapist Assistant
QA	Quality Assurance
QI	Quality Improvement
RN	Registered Nurse
SLP	Speech-Language Pathology
ST	Speech Therapy
TB	Tuberculosis
TV	Television
VA	Veterans Administration

Appendix C

EDUCATIONAL RESOURCES

Caring
228 7th Street SE
Washington, DC 20003–4306
Published monthly by the National Association for Home Care (NAHC)

HHNA Forum
437 Twin Bay Drive
Pensacola, FL 32534
A bimonthly newsletter published by the Home Healthcare Nurses Association

Home Care Nurse News
P.O. Box 391
Westerville, OH 43086–0391
A monthly publication by Marrelli and Associates

Home Health Focus
Mosby-Yearbook, Inc.
11830 Westline Industrial Dr.
St. Louis, MO 63146–3318
A monthly newsletter for home care professionals

Home Healthcare Nurse
12107 Insurance Way
Hagerstown, MD 21740
Published monthly by Lippincott-Raven Publishers

(continued)

Educational Resources *(continued)*

Nurseweek
1156–C Aster Ave.
Sunnyvale, CA 94086
Published biweekly by NURSE WEEK Publishing, Inc.

Nursing 96
1111 Bethlehem Pike, Box 908
Springhouse, PA 19477
Published monthly by Springhouse Corporation

RN
5 Paragon Drive
Montvale, NJ 07645
Published monthly by Medical Economics Publishing Company

Appendix D

TOOLS OF THE TRADE

Items	*Details*	*Specifics*
Nursing bag	*Contents:* • liquid soap • paper towels • towelettes • alcohol wipes • stethoscope • sphygmomanometer • penlight • measuring tape • gloves • tongue blades • cotton balls • 4 x 4 & 2 x 2 tape • Band-Aids® • tourniquet • hemostat • bandage scissors • thermometers • disposable resuscitation mask • face shield • disposable apron	• The better bags are made of waterproof material • Items can be organized by categories using small clear plastic bags • Backpacks are also suitable • To prevent theft, do not leave the bag in view when the car is unattended
Reference books	Drug book Home care manual	• Available at specialty book stores

(continued)

Tools of the Trade *(continued)*

Items	*Details*	*Specifics*
Lists	*Phone numbers:* • co-workers' beepers • ambulances • In Home Diagnostic Services (x-ray, EKG, labs, blood gases lab) • hospitals • medical equipment suppliers • IV vendors • coroner • senior services • MDs, podiatrists who make house calls	• A compact electronic organizer can be used to keep all the phone numbers at hand
Beeper		• Usually provided by agency
Other items	Maps	• Choose easy-to-read ones; local street atlases have larger type and are very suitable • Laminated maps have longer wear and tear resistance • Keep one map in the car, and one at the office
	Self-stick notes	
Sharps container		• Usually provided by agency; when ¾ full, dispose of as per agency's protocol
Coin purse		• The best ones come equipped with an alarm, to save parking tickets

(continued)

Tools of the Trade *(continued)*

Items	*Details*	*Specifics*
Cellular phone		• Can be expensive if agency does not provide
Laptop computer		• Limited use now; wave of the future

Appendix E

YOUR CAR

YOUR CAR (AS TRANSPORTATION)

Goal	*Actions*
Most useful features	• Size: economy, and mini-compact • Air bags • Radio/cassette/CD player • Air conditioner • Keyless lock • Car phone
Ways to minimize repairs	• Check oil level each time you purchase gasoline • Change oil regularly • Keep engine in good repair • Keep tires at the proper inflation pressure • Protect tires from rubbing against the curb when parallel parking • Familiarize yourself with the normal sounds of your car
Ways to cut operating costs	• Pump own gas • Use proper gasoline octane • Do not keep engine idling • Drive a smaller car

(continued)

Goal	Actions
	• Scooter: *Advantage:* size, ease of parking *Disadvantage:* little protection against the elements
Emergency ready	• Keep an emergency auto kit in trunk • Keep spare tire in good condition • Subscribe to a road emergency service

YOUR CAR (AS OFFICE)

Goal	Actions
Facilitate work	• Organize the interior to access items quickly • Place maps, pens, pencils, sunglasses, and water bottle in a basket on the floor on the passenger side • Keep handy in the car a supply of the forms most often used

YOUR CAR (AS CLASSROOM)

Goals	Actions
• Make driving time more constructive • Break monotony	• Listen to recordings of: medical subjects, languages, foreign medical terminology, inservices presented at work, continuing education, books, public radio, inspirational or self-improvement tapes • Silence: thinking or problem-solving time

Appendix F

OCCUPATIONAL HAZARDS: PREVENTION

Hazards	*Actions*
• Pain in shoulders from carrying too heavy a nursing bag	• Review contents of nursing bag regularly and remove accumulated, unnecessary supplies to lighten the load and reduce pressure on the shoulders
• Pain in hands from increased writing time	• Add a "comfort grip" to a pen (small rubber cushion to absorb pressure) • Keep arm level to writing surface; raise or lower chair, if necessary
• Neck and back pain from frequent parking and increased driving time	• When turning neck to parallel park, push the opposite leg forward to prevent over twisting of neck • Use car mirrors as much as possible • Add small pillow to lumbar area • Consider using a seat pad made of rounded beads; it facilitates pivoting and reduces fatigue • When charting in the car, change position frequently; make sure the seat is pushed back as far as possible to allow maximum mobility

REFERENCES

Albrecht, M. N. (1990). The Albrecht nursing model for home health care: implications for research, practice, and education. *Public Health Nursing, 7*, pp. 118–126.

American Nurses Association. (1985). Code for nurses. Kansas City, MO: Author.

American Nurses Association (1985). Code for nurses with interpretive statements, p. 3. Washington, DC: Author.

American Nurses Association. (1986). *Standards of community health nursing practice.* Washington, DC: Author.

American Nurses Association. (1986). *Standards of home health nursing practice.* Kansas City, MO: Author.

American Nurses Association. (1993, May). Sexual harassment: It's against the law. Washington, DC.

Anglin, L. T. (1992). Caseload management. *Home Healthcare Nurse, 10*(3), pp. 26–31.

Batey, M. V., & Lewis, F. M. (1982). Clarifying autonomy and accountability in nursing service: Part 1. *The Journal of Nursing Administration XII*(9), pp. 13–18.

Blue Cross of California (1993). Documentation of management and evaluation of care plan. *Bulletin 346*. Oxnard, CA: Author.

Brault, G. L. (1991). Home care is the place to be in the '90's. *California Nursing, 87*(10) p. 8.

Ceslowitz, S. B., & Loreti, S. T. (1991). Easing the transition from hospital nursing to home care: A research study. *Home Healthcare Nurse, 9*(4), pp. 32–35.

Collins, S. S., & Henderson, M. (1991). Autonomy: Part of the nursing role? *Nursing Forum, 26*(2), pp. 23–28.

Faherty, B. (1990). Home care under Medicare in the '90s. *NurseWeek/North*, pp. 12–14.

Foreman, J. T. (1993). Continuous quality improvement in home care. *Caring, XII*(10), pp. 32–37.

Gabe, M., & Gill-Forney, B. (1993). Reaching for the ideal in home care. *Home Healthcare Nurse, 11*(6), pp. 30–33.

Gilbert, N. J. (1992). Supervision of home health paraprofessionals. *Caring, XL*(4), pp. 10–14.

Greve, P. (1991). Advance directives—What the new law means for you. *RN, 54*(11), pp. 63–67.

Harris, M. D. (1994). *Handbook of home health care administration*. Gaithersburg, MD: Aspen Publishers.

Humphrey, C. J. (1994). *Home care nursing handbook.* Gaithersburg, MD: Aspen Publishers.

Humphrey, C. J., & Milone-Nuzzo, P. (1996). *Orientation to home care nursing.* Gaithersburg, MD: Aspen Publishers.

Jaffe, M. S., & Skidmore-Roth, L. (1993). *Home health nursing care plans* (2nd ed.) St. Louis, MO: Mosby-Year Book.

Joint Commission on Accreditation of Healthcare Organizations. (1995b). Accreditation manual for home care, Volume 2: Scoring guidelines, pp. 290–291. Management of Human Resources section. Oakbrook Terrace, IL: Author.

Liebermann, A. R. (1990). *Community home health nursing.* Springhouse, PA: Springhouse.

MacLaren, E. (1994). Basics of managed care. *NurseWeek,* pp. 10–11.

McHann, M. (1995). *What every home health nurse needs to know.* New York, NY: Springer Publishing Company.

Messner, R. L., & Gardner, S. S. (1993). Start with the medicine cabinet. *RN, 56*(1), pp. 51–53.

National Hospice Organization (1984). *The basics of Hospice* (pamphlet). Arlington, VA: Author.

National Association for Home Care (1993). *Homecare bill of rights.* Washington, DC: Author.

National Association for Home Care (1995). *Basic statistics about home care 1995* (p. 1). Washington, DC: Author.

Personal vigilance: A safety guide for women (and men). (1992). *USAA Aide Magazine, 23*(1), pp. 6–7.

San Francisco Police Department. *SAFE, a community crime prevention program, Safety for older adults* (pamphlet). San Francisco, CA: Author.

Thobaben, M. (1993). Sexual harassment. *Home Healthcare Nurse, 11*(6), pp. 66–67.

U.S. Department of Health and Human Services, Medicare Coverage of Services (April 1996). Health insurance manual–11, transmittal revision No. 277. Washington, DC: Health Care Financing Administration.

BIBLIOGRAPHY

9-1-1: Know the number, know when to use it. *SAFE A community crime prevention program.* (pamphlet) San Francisco, CA: San Francisco Police Department.

Allen, S. A. (1994). Medicare case management. *Home Healthcare Nurse, 12,* pp. 21–27.

American Nurses Association. (1992). *A statement on the scope of home health nursing practice.* Washington, DC: Author.

Barkauskas, V. H. (1994). Case management within home care. *Home Healthcare Nurse, 12,* p. 8.

Bates, B. (1993). *Physical examination and history taking.* Philadelphia, PA: Lippincott.

Batey, M. V., & Lewis, F. M. (1982). Clarifying autonomy and accountability in nursing service: Part 2. *The Journal of Nursing Administration, XII*(10), pp. 10–15.

Belanus, A., & Hunt, P. (1993). When orientation is not enough. *Home Healthcare Nurse, 10*(6), pp. 36–40.

Belcher, A. E. (1992). *Cancer nursing.* St. Louis, MO: Mosby-Year Book.

Board of Registered Nursing. (1992). *Nursing practice act.* Sacramento, CA: State of California Department of Consumer Affairs.

Boutotte, J. (1993). T. B.: The second time around . . . and how you can help to control it. *Nursing93, 87*(10), pp. 42–49.

Bower, K. A. (1992). *Case management by nurses.* Washington, DC: American Nurses Association.

Brady, B. (1994, May). How I was sexually harassed, and why you don't have to be. *Nursing94, 24*(5), pp. 52–56.

Brent, N. J. (1993). Delegation and supervision of patient care. *Home Healthcare Nurse, 11*(4), pp. 7–8.

Burbach, C. A. L., Conrad, M. B., Lindsay, L. (1991). Issues in home health nursing education. *Home Healthcare Nurse, 9*(4), pp. 22–28.

Canfield, J. (1989). *How to build high self-esteem.* Chicago, IL: Nightingale-Conant.

Carr, P. (1991). A whole different world. *Home Healthcare Nurse, 9*(4), pp. 6–7.

Collopy, B., Dubler, N., & Zuckerman, C. (1990). The ethics of home care: Autonomy and accommodation. *Hastings Center Report, 20*(2), pp. 1–16.

Cooke, M. K., & Brodrick, T. M. (1994). Critical pathways. In M. Dattarris (Ed.), *Hand-book of home health care administration* (pp. 309–319). Gaithersburg, MD: Aspen Publishers.

de Savorgnani, A., Haring, R. C., & Galloway, S. (1992). Caught in the middle. *Caring, XI*(9), pp. 12–16.

Ebersole, P., & Hess, P. (1994). *Toward healthy aging* (4th ed.). St. Louis, MO: C. V. Mosby.

Ferri, R. S. (1994). *Care planning for the older adult*. Philadelphia, PA: W. B. Saunders.

Forsyth, D., & Cannady, J. (1981). Preventing and alleviating staff burnout through a group. *Journal of Psychosocial Nursing and Mental Health Services, 19*, pp. 33–38.

Frawley, K. A. (1994). Confidentiality in the computer age. *RN 57*(7), pp. 59–60.

Giger, J. N., & Davidhizar, R. E. (1991). *Transcultural nursing: Assessment and intervention*. St. Louis, MO: Mosby-Year Book.

Glover, D., King, M., Green, C., & Shults, A. (1993). The patient care team advantage. *Caring, XII*(10), pp. 40–42.

Guillory, B. A., & Riggin, O. Z. (1991). Developing a nursing staff support group model. *Clinical Nurse Specialist, 5*(3), pp. 170–173.

Harris, M. D., & Schmidt, D. (1993). Supervision of home care aides. *Home Healthcare Nurse, 11*(4), pp. 51–53.

Harris, M. D., & Yuan, J. (1991). Educating and orienting nurses for home healthcare. *Home Healthcare Nurse, 9*(4), pp. 9–14.

Haw, M. N., & Durbin-Lafferty, E. (1984). Improving nursing morale in a climate of cost containment. *The Journal of Nursing Administration, 14*(10), pp. 8–14.

Health care reform: Home health is part of the solution. (1993, February 19). *CAHSAH bulletin*. Sacramento, CA.

Hedrick, S. C., & Inui, T. S. (1986). The effectiveness and cost of home care: An information synthesis. *Health Services Research, 20*(6), pp. 851–880.

Home Care Financing Administration (1989). *Medicare home health agency manual Publication 11*. Washington, DC: Author.

Humphrey, C. J., & Milone-Nuzzo, P. (1993). Home care nursing orientation model: Justification and structure. *Home Healthcare Nurse, 10*(3), pp. 18–22.

Hussar, D. (1994). *Modell's Drugs in current use and new drugs* (40th ed.). New York, NY: Springer Publishing Company.

Jackson, J. E., & Johnson, E. A. (1988). *Patient education in home care: A practical guide to effective teaching and documentation*. Rockville, MD: Aspen Publishers.

Jaffe, M. (1991). Geriatric nursing care plans. El Paso, TX: Skidmore Roth Publications.

Kirkis, E. J. (1993). Home health/public health/visiting nurse returning to our past. *Home Healthcare Nurse, 11*(5), pp. 9–13.

Kluckowski, J. C. (1992). Solving medication noncompliance in home care. *Caring, XI*(11), pp. 34–41.

Leimnetzer, M. J., Ryan, D. A., & Niemann, V. G. (1993). The hospital-visiting nurse association partnership. *JONA, 23*(11), pp. 20–23.

Lipkin, G. B., & Cohen, R. G. (1992). *Effective approaches to patients' behavior* (4th ed.). New York, NY: Springer Publishing Company.

London, F. (1995). Teach your patients faster better. *Nursing95, 25*(8), pp. 68–70.

Lueckenotte, A. G. (1990). *Pocket guide to gerontologic assessment*. St. Louis, MO: C. V. Mosby.

MacDonald, S. A., Brodie, K., Winn, S., Wilhardt, L., & Williams, T. (1992). Reimbursement warfare: Who loses? *Home Healthcare Nurse, 9*(6), pp. 9–12.

Marrelli, T. M. (1994). *Handbook of home health standards and documentation guidelines for reimbursement* (2nd ed.). St. Louis, MO: Mosby-Year Book.

McCarthy, T., Gunther, W., & Hoffman, C. L. (1994). *The nursing assistant*. Englewood Cliffs, NJ: Regents/Prentice Hall.

Meyers, D. (1989). *Client teaching guides for home health care*. Rockville, MD: Aspen Publishers.

Mezey, M. D., Rauckhorst, L. M., & Stokes, S. A. (1993). *Health assessment of the older individual* (2nd ed.). New York, NY: Springer Publishing Company.

Milone-Nuzzo, P., & Humphrey, C. J. (1993). Home care nursing orientation model: Content and strategies. *Home Healthcare Nurse, 10*(6), pp. 24–30.

Molloy, S. P. (1994). Defining case management. *Home Healthcare Nurse, 12*(3), pp. 51–54.

National League for Nursing. (1980). *Ethical issues in nursing and nursing education*. New York, NY: Author.

National League for Nursing. (1986). *Case studies in nursing theory* (P. W. Fry, Ed.). New York, NY: Author.

National uniformity for paraprofessional title, qualifications, and supervision. (1992). *Caring, XI*(4), pp. 4–9.

Neck owner's manual (1985). Daly City, CA: Krames Communications.

Norbeck, J. S., Lindsey, A. M., & Carrieri, V. L. (1981). The development of an instrument to measure social support. *Nursing Research, 30*(5), pp. 264–269.

Nornhold, P. (1994). Hospital restructuring: How to cope with the changes. *Nursing94, 24*(9), pp. 47–49.

O'Reilly, D. P. M. (1982). Toward autonomy of the nursing profession. *Nursing Leadership, 5*(3), pp. 18–22.

OSHA mandates AIDS protection. (1992). *Caring, XI*(2), pp. 40–42.

Otto, S. E. (1994). *Oncology nursing* (2nd ed.) St. Louis, MO: Mosby-Year Book.

Rhoads, C., Dean, J., Cason, C., & Blaylock, A. (1993). Comprehensive discharge planning. *Home Healthcare Nurse, 10*(6), pp. 13–18.

Rice, R., & Jorden, J. U. (1992). Infection control education for home care aides. *Caring, XL*(4), pp. 54–59.

Rice, R. (1996). Home health nursing practice; concepts & application (2nd ed.). St. Louis, MO: Mosby-Year Book.

Roberts, S. L. (1990). Achieving professional autonomy through nursing diagnosis and nursing DRGs. *Nursing Administration Quarterly, 14*(4), pp. 54–60.

Rogers, J. L., & Maurizio, S. J. (1993). Prevalence of sexual harassment among rural community care workers. *Home Healthcare Nurse, 11*(4), pp. 37–40.

Rogers-Seidl, F. F. (1991). *Geriatric nursing care plans*. St. Louis, MO: Mosby-Year Book.

Sheldon, J. E. (1994). Combating infection: 25 tips on hand washing. *Nursing94, 24*(1), p. 20.

Sherry, D. (1993). Cost effectiveness and home care: Myth or reality? *Home Healthcare Nurse, 10*(1), pp. 27–29.

Singleton, E. K., & Nail, F. C. (1984). Role clarification: A prerequisite to autonomy. *The Journal of Nursing Administration, 14*(10), pp. 17–22.

Smith, F. D. (1991). *The driving skills book*. 6. How to be a smarter driver (booklet). *Shell Oil Company*.

Stanhope, M., & Knollmueller, R. N. (1992). *Handbook of community and home health nursing*. St. Louis, MO: Mosby-Year Book.

Stanhope, M., & Lancaster, J. (1992). *Community health nursing* (3rd ed.). St. Louis, MO: Mosby-Year Book.

Stanhope, M. & Lancaster, J. (1993). *Quick reference to community health nursing*. St. Louis, MO: Mosby-Year Book.

Stewart, J. E. (1979). *Home health care*. St. Louis, MO: C. V. Mosby.

Twardon, C., Cherry, C., & Gartner, M. (1992). Home care aide evaluation: Assuring competency quality. *Caring, 11*(6), pp. 16–20.

Twardon, C., Gartner, M., & Cherry, C. (1993). A competency achievement orientation program. *JONA, 23*(7/8), pp. 20–25.

Van Blarcom, K. (1993). Home care standards: A necessity for quality. *Caring, XII*(10), pp. 77–80.

Wagnild, G., & Grupp, K. (1991). Major stressors among elderly home care clients. *Home Healthcare Nurse, 9*(4), pp. 15–21.

Weber, J. (1991). *Nurse's handbook of health assessment*. Philadelphia, PA: J. B. Lippincott.

INDEX

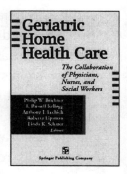